Library of Congress Control Number: 2022938350

First Printing, 2022

Publisher: Dustin Sullivan

Acquisitions Editor: Emily Hatch

Development Editor: Rebecca Senninger

Cover Designer: Rebecca Batchelor

Interior Design/Page Layout: Rebecca Batchelor

Indexer: Larry Sweazy

Managing Editor: Carla Hall

Publications Specialist: Todd Lothery

Project Editor: Rebecca Senninger

Copy Editor: Erin Geile

Proofreader: Todd Lothery

T0243372

Dedication

We would like to dedicate this book to all the patients and families who have inspired these case studies and who have allowed us to serve, care for, and walk alongside them during their challenging healthcare situations. We are better nurses because of you. Thank you for your stories and making this possible.

ETHICAL CASE STUDIES

Solving Dilemmas in Everyday Practice

FOR ADVANCED PRACTICE NURSES

Amber L. Vermeesch, PhD, MSN, RN, FNP-C, FACSM, FNAP, ANEF

Patricia H. Cox, DNP, MPH, MN, BSN, RN

Inga M. Giske, DNP, MSN, RN, PMHNP-BC, PMH-BC, NE-BC

Katherine M. Roberts, DNP, BSN, RN, FNP-C

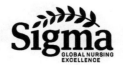

Sigma
GLOBAL NURSING
EXCELLENCE

Copyright © 2023 by Sigma Theta Tau International Honor Society of Nursing

All rights reserved. This book is protected by copyright. No part of it may be reproduced, stored in a retrieval system, or transmitted in any form or by any means, electronic, mechanical, photocopying, recording, or otherwise, without written permission from the publisher. Any trademarks, service marks, design rights, or similar rights that are mentioned, used, or cited in this book are the property of their respective owners. Their use here does not imply that you may use them for a similar or any other purpose.

This book is not intended to be a substitute for the medical advice of a licensed medical professional. The author and publisher have made every effort to ensure the accuracy of the information contained within at the time of its publication and shall have no liability or responsibility to any person or entity regarding any loss or damage incurred, or alleged to have incurred, directly or indirectly, by the information contained in this book. The author and publisher make no warranties, express or implied, with respect to its content, and no warranties may be created or extended by sales representatives or written sales materials. The author and publisher have no responsibility for the consistency or accuracy of URLs and content of third-party websites referenced in this book.

Sigma Theta Tau International Honor Society of Nursing (Sigma) is a nonprofit organization whose mission is developing nurse leaders anywhere to improve healthcare everywhere. Founded in 1922, Sigma has more than 135,000 active members in over 100 countries and territories. Members include practicing nurses, instructors, researchers, policymakers, entrepreneurs, and others. Sigma's more than 540 chapters are located at more than 700 institutions of higher education throughout Armenia, Australia, Botswana, Brazil, Canada, Colombia, Croatia, England, Eswatini, Ghana, Hong Kong, Ireland, Israel, Italy, Jamaica, Japan, Jordan, Kenya, Lebanon, Malawi, Mexico, the Netherlands, Nigeria, Pakistan, Philippines, Portugal, Puerto Rico, Scotland, Singapore, South Africa, South Korea, Sweden, Taiwan, Tanzania, Thailand, the United States, and Wales. Learn more at www.sigmanursing.org.

Sigma Theta Tau International
550 West North Street
Indianapolis, IN, USA 46202

To request a review copy for course adoption, order additional books, buy in bulk, or purchase for corporate use, contact Sigma Marketplace at 888.654.4968 (US/Canada toll-free), +1.317.687.2256 (International), or solutions@sigmamarketplace.org.

To request author information, or for speaker or other media requests, contact Sigma Marketing at 888.634.7575 (US/Canada toll-free) or +1.317.634.8171 (International).

ISBN: 9781646480906
EPUB ISBN: 9781646480913
PDF ISBN: 9781646480920

Praise for *Ethical Case Studies for Advanced Practice Nurses*

"I am decidedly impressed by Drs. Vermeesch, Cox, Giske, and Roberts' new book, *Ethical Case Studies for Advanced Practice Nurses*. I wish this workbook would have been available for preparation for practice when I was a student in my own FNP/DNP program, as many of these case studies feel as if they were lifted from my own encounters. I plan on using this text with students I precept in my own practice in the future. What a wonderful way to see advanced practice nursing as neither black nor white but instead as a myriad of colors in which to hone principled and just care as our Code of Nursing intends."

–Laurel Hallock-Koppelman, DNP, APRN, FNP-C
Assistant Professor, School of Medicine, Oregon Health and Science University

"Ethical Case Studies for Advanced Practice Nurses gracefully guides readers through the sorts of ethically complex cases that keep us all up at night. Infused with wisdom and clarity, this textbook is a must-read for APRNs of all practice environments and levels of experience. As a clinical ethicist, I was deeply impressed— although not surprised, as it is authored by four powerhouses in the field—by how much I learned within the pages of this book."

–Kayla Tabari-House, MBE, RN, HEC-C
Clinical Ethicist, Providence St. Joseph Health

"Teaching ethics to graduate nursing students can be challenging because so many students enter into discussions with preconceived notions about how ethics are relegated to legal or philosophical debates, or their only exposure to ethics is through cut-and-dried lectures. The beauty of this text is that it provides the reader with real-world, common-sense examples of the types of ethical challenges often faced by those who practice in advanced practice roles. The authors masterfully created cases grounded in reality that bring the ethical concepts of the ANA Code alive in ways that allow for nuanced conversation and engaged learning. Perfect for flipped classrooms and other student participative methodologies, this book would be easy to incorporate into any advanced practice clinical course designed for students who will work in community-based settings."

–Dawn Garzon, PhD, CPNP-PC, PMHS, FAANP, FAAN
Behavioral Health Nurse Practitioner
St. Louis Children's Hospital

"An excellent resource for both new and experienced practitioners. The case studies in this book help nurses recognize that some everyday clinical encounters represent ethical dilemmas that can leave the practitioner feeling uncomfortable. The book presents a wide range of situations that any practitioner may encounter and offers a framework for systematically reviewing the problem and developing viable solutions."

–Mary A Kozy, PhD, RN
Professor (retired), University of Portland School of Nursing
Former Dean, Linfield University School of Nursing

"As historical, emerging, and not-yet-imagined healthcare concerns challenge our nation and world, nurses will continue to lead the efforts to accompany the most vulnerable in their times of uncertainty and need. This book is an excellent tool to guide advanced practice registered nurses and their collaborators in healthcare education into conversations about ethical action within the complex challenges of their work."

–Daniel McGinty, EdD
Dundon-Berchtold Institute for Moral Formation & Applied Ethics
University of Portland

"Ethical discernment and problem-solving present an especially difficult challenge for nurses. This book provides common clinical situations that advanced practice nurses face with a helpful framework to guide the nurse in reflection and discussing with colleagues. Faculty will find these case studies useful in teaching ethical reasoning, and consultation groups of clinicians can use them to clarify similar situations they are confronting. Kudos to the authors in providing timely and essential case studies."

–Barbara J. Limandri, PhD, PMHCNS-BC, PMHNP

"Ethical decisions are often a point of professional and personal angst in nursing practice across all levels of academic preparation. They can be particularly troublesome in advanced practice, where clinicians are faced with complex issues that require consideration of a multitude of factors in an often brief patient/family encounter. The cases offered in this publication are reflective of the dilemmas occurring every day in APRN practice in both primary and acute settings and provide a much-needed resource that can be used to enrich and expand our preparation of APRNs to care for patients and families. Graduate programs can use these cases across the curriculum, while professional organizations and employers can use them to stimulate ongoing professional development of our APRN workforce and critical conversations that support and improve both the patient and APRN experience of care. I wholeheartedly endorse this book and encourage its use as we continue to seek best practices in educating our next generation of APRNs."

–Mary Koithan, PhD, RN, CNS-BC, FAAN
Professor and Dean
Washington State University College of Nursing

Acknowledgments

We would like to acknowledge the opportunities and financial support provided by the Dundon-Berchtold Institute at the University of Portland and, particularly, the unwavering encouragement of Dr. Daniel McGinty. Additionally, we would like to acknowledge Drs. David McAnulty and Annie Tubman for their aid in providing guidance on several case studies based on their collective years of practice. Furthermore, Dr. Rahul Lauhan and clinical ethicists, Dr. Nick Kockler and Kevin Dirksen, are acknowledged for their unwavering support through numerous ethical conundrums.

About the Authors

Amber L. Vermeesch, PhD, MSN, RN, FNP-C, FACSM, FNAP, ANEF, has been a practicing family nurse practitioner since 2006. She has spent most of her practice serving underinsured and vulnerable populations. She completed her master's in nursing at Vanderbilt University School of Nursing. She earned her PhD in nursing science from the University of Miami in 2011, where she focused on reducing healthcare disparities among Latino populations using multiple methodologies, including participatory photography. She joined the University of Portland as an Associate Professor in 2014, teaching in both graduate and undergraduate programs, and served as the Director of Research and Scholarship. She became a certified nurse educator in 2017. In 2022, Vermeesch was inducted as a Fellow in the National League for Nursing Academy of Nursing Education; in 2020, she became a Fellow in the American College of Sports Medicine as well as Distinguished Practitioner and Fellow in the National Academies of Practice. Her overall area of expertise is wellness, both physical and emotional. In 2022, she became the Department Chair for Family and Community Nursing at the University of North Carolina at Greensboro. Her investigations have concentrated on physical activity and integrated health among vulnerable populations. Additionally, she explores risk factors related to stress reduction and health promotion among undergraduates and graduate students as well as faculty and staff. Patricia Cox (2014–2015) and Vermeesch (2015–2016) laid the initial foundations for this workbook through individual fellowship projects in the Application of Ethics provided by the Dundon-Berchtold Institute. All four main authors—Cox, Vermeesch, Inga Giske, and Katherine Roberts— participated in the Ethics Curriculum Fellowship 2019–2020 provided by the Dundon-Berchtold Institute to develop those projects into this workbook.

Patricia H. Cox, DNP, MPH, MN, BSN, RN, recently retired as the Director of Doctoral Nursing Education & Practice at the School of Nursing at the University of Portland. Her long career in nursing took her from the bedside as an Army nurse to working as a public health nurse with migrant farmworkers and then Lao refugees in Thailand. Along the way, she advanced her education while caring for HIV/AIDS patients as a nurse practitioner in the early days of the epidemic. Later she provided primary care to Native American and Hispanic populations in a community clinic in Los Angeles. Always supportive of nursing education, Cox served as adjunct faculty in several nursing programs prior to relocating to Portland to teach full time and prepare the next generation of nurse practitioners in the DNP Program at the University of Portland.

Inga M. Giske, DNP, MSN, RN, PMHNP-BC, PMH-BC, NE-BC, serves as a psychiatric nurse practitioner on the Psychiatric Consult-Liaison service at Providence St. Vincent Medical Center. She provides psychiatric evaluation and treatment recommendations for patients during their medical admission while also providing education and support to professional staff, nursing, and ancillary care team members. In addition, she serves as a preceptor to nurse practitioner students, medical students, and internal medicine residents. Her nursing career has spanned from bedside nursing to regional leadership in acute inpatient psychiatric units and psychiatric emergency departments. She implemented evidence-based practice changes in both acute inpatient and psychiatric settings to reduce falls and violence and improve patient and caregiver satisfaction. Giske works to improve knowledge regarding mental health conditions and reduce stigma through education of nurses, other healthcare providers, and her community. She has been adjunct faculty at the University of Portland, teaching undergraduate psychiatric nursing. She provides competency-based suicide assessment training to nurses both locally and nationally. Lastly, she has served as a trainer to local law enforcement in her community, educating both new recruits and experienced officers on mental health, crisis intervention, and de-escalation for the past six years.

Katherine Roberts, DNP, BSN, RN, FNP-C, is a recent DNP graduate from the University of Portland. Although new to the DNP role, she has an extensive background as a bachelor-prepared registered nurse. After graduating from Linfield College in 2004, Roberts has practiced in various settings, including the Childhood Development and Rehabilitation Center at Doernbecher Children's Hospital and Neonatal Intensive Care Unit at Randell's Children's hospital in Portland. More recently and for most of her career, she worked for Northwest Primary Care Group. Her experience with patients extends to all ages and stages of life and various levels of care, from a nursing assistant working with developmentally and physically disabled children to a bedside nurse working with well and ill newborn and preterm infants. Eventually, she found her passion in family medicine, working with patients of all ages, including pregnant women. As a nursing leader, Roberts worked as a charge nurse for many years before eventually taking a more administrative role writing policy and procedure and creating a unique nursing and patient education program. In May 2018, she lost her friend and mentor, Dr. Margret "Peggy" McNichol, who began her career as a nurse and always taught her to strive to make the world a better place, one problem and patient at a time. Thus, Roberts decided to advance her education, get back to direct patient care, and continue making a difference for the patients and profession of nursing as a doctorally prepared nurse practitioner.

Contributing Authors

Larlene Dunsmuir, DNP, FNP, ANP-C, has been a nurse practitioner since 1993 and maintains a clinical practice, teaches as adjunct faculty at the University of Portland School of Nursing, and is employed as the Director of Professional Services by the Oregon Nurses Association, where she oversees the continuing nursing education program. Dunsmuir brings a wealth of experience and knowledge of nursing practice, policy, and education to her work. She has practiced in neurology, family medicine, and urgent care. From 1995–2005, she co-owned a family care clinic with another nurse practitioner. One of the things she is most proud of is participating in creating a nurse practitioner telehealth practice in 2012 that now serves patients in several states. She received her BS in nursing in 1985 from the University of Portland (UP). She returned to UP to complete her master's degree in nursing with a focus in adult health nurse practitioner in 1993 and a family nurse practitioner post-master's certificate program in 2000. She completed her doctor of nursing practice in 2014 at Chatham University in Pittsburgh.

Kristine Dukart-Harrington, DNP, RN, AGNP-C, ACHPN, is an assistant professor and chair of the Adult-Gerontology Primary Care Nurse Practitioner track at the University of Portland School of Nursing. She has practiced in hospice and palliative care for most of her 10-year nursing career, most recently as an oncology palliative care provider at Providence Portland Medical Center. She earned her doctor of nursing practice degree and post-master's certificate as an Adult-Gerontology Primary Care Nurse Practitioner at Duke University School of Nursing. She is honored and humbled to be present with people who are navigating the uncertainties of living with advanced illness. She hopes to empower and inspire her students to become skilled communicators, fierce advocates, and thoughtful caregivers.

Norma Lubeck, DO, is an anesthesiologist with experiences in trauma, OB/GYN, and general anesthesia. She received her DO degree at the College of Osteopathic Medicine of the Pacific, Pomona, California in 1996. As a Colonel in the Army Reserves Medical Corps, she deployed to Bosnia-Herzegovina and to Iraq for Operation Enduring Freedom. Prior to medical school and residency, Lubeck was a CRNA and an Army Reservist in the Nurse Corps and deployed to the Middle East during Desert Shield/Storm. She received her BSN (1981) and MSN (1985) at California State University, Long Beach. She was an Adjunct Professor at the CSULB-affiliated Kaiser Permanente School of Nurse Anesthesia. Prior to teaching, she provided anesthesia care to patients at a large Los Angeles County hospital serving low-income and underinsured populations. As a clinical provider, Lubeck has experienced the complex and compounded problems associated with anesthesia care. Ethical dilemmas reach beyond direct patient and loved ones' needs to involve the bedside nurse, attending physician, hospital administrator, and risk management office. She retired from anesthesia practice in 2022.

Maren Nelson, DNP, FNP-C, is an Assistant Professor and the Chair of the FNP track at the University of Portland. She is passionate about family practice, primary care, and the role of lifestyle medicine in the prevention and management of chronic illness. Nursing is a second career for her. She earned her BSN in 2009 and her DNP in 2015, both from the University of Portland.

Joanne Olsen, PhD, RN, CPHQ, CPSO, held her most recent position in health system board governance. She has also held positions in hospital administration, research, academic leadership, and academic teaching. Her governance responsibilities included overseeing the big picture in meeting the health system mission and long-term strategy. The health system served a region of over 80,000 square miles. In Olsen's healthcare operations roles, she has coordinated the delivery of healthcare services, balancing the coaction of quality, safety, legal, political, ethical, and financial complexities in healthcare delivery practice and approaches. Olsen has held healthcare leadership positions in academic, community, and critical access hospitals. In academia, she taught undergraduate and graduate courses that explored ethical behavior standards, ethics, and decision-making using examples from contemporary practices in the healthcare industry.

Additional Book Resources

To download a free sample chapter and other book-related materials, visit the *Ethical Case Studies for Advanced Practice Nurses* page on the Sigma Repository via the link or QR code.

http://hdl.handle.net/10755/22743

Table of Contents

It should be no surprise that today's healthcare technologies have come at a rapid pace and that the patchwork quilt of our healthcare system has struggled to keep up to provide safe, affordable, and accessible healthcare to all. Nurses have met the challenge by increasing their knowledge base and use of technology, and they recently demonstrated their dedication during the COVID-19 pandemic.

For an amazing 22 years, a Gallup poll has consistently reported that nursing is the most honest and ethical profession. This is fitting as we celebrate the 202nd anniversary of Florence Nightingale's birth, the acknowledged founder of modern nursing. Evidenced-based practice began with Nightingale, and she dedicated her life to improving healthcare, preventing disease, and advocating safe treatment for all. For years I taught evidenced-based practice—the process of collecting, processing, and implementing research findings to improve clinical practice and patient outcomes. By using this approach, nurses provide high-quality, cost-effective care. This is an essential element of all nursing school curricula. Of course, providing ethical care is a cornerstone of that practice. Dilemmas occur when the choice is not clear-cut on what to do or the options are not ideal. Quality care, clinical outcomes, and relationships may suffer as a consequence.

In my many years of teaching and in my role as Associate Dean for Graduate Programs, I saw how faculty and graduate and undergraduate students struggled with ethical dilemmas that arose in their clinical practice. *Ethical Case Studies for Advanced Practice Nurses* is a workbook written by nurse practitioners and seasoned nurse practitioner faculty who completed fellowships in applied ethics offered through the Dundon-Berchtold Institute at the University of Portland. Their fellowships began with concerns that graduate advanced practice students were unable to identify such quandaries in their clinical experiences. This book captures key conflicts common to advanced practice nursing and allows nurses to reflect on and think through the ethical, moral, and legal aspects of each dilemma using a public health framework.

The authors have written a powerful resource for preparing advanced practice nurses, DNP students, and practicing nurse practitioners to face ethical conundrums that arise in their clinical practice. The content is challenging, and the real-world case studies make this book essential for educating advanced practice students.

Both students and faculty teaching in advanced practice programs will find this educational tool a "must-have" for their personal library.

–Susan Stillwell, DNP, RN, ANEF, FAAN
Former Associate Dean for Graduate Programs (retired)
University of Portland, Portland, Oregon, USA

Introduction

"Let us never consider ourselves finished nurses . . .
we must be learning all of our lives."

–Florence Nightingale

Significant changes have occurred in the healthcare environment over the last five years. Despite attempts to dismantle the Affordable Care Act (ACA), an increasing number of individuals are receiving healthcare according to the US Department of Health and Human Services. Its June 2021 report announced that 31 million Americans are now covered with health insurance through the ACA (HHS.gov, 2021).

The National Academies of Sciences, Engineering and Medicine have called for every American to have a primary caregiver (Levey, 2021). The Academies recognize that the backbone in our healthcare system to providing high quality care is through primary care (Levey, 2021). To do this, more nurse practitioners, pharmacists, and mental health providers are needed in primary care and community clinics (Community Catalyst, n.d.). For decades, advanced practice registered nurses (APRNs) have delivered high-quality specialty and primary care and have improved access to those seeking care (Schiff, 2012).

For 20 years in a row, Gallup has conducted its poll on Honesty and Ethics and nurses continue to rate as the most trusted profession (Saad, 2022). Eighty-one percent of Americans rated nurses as trustworthy above all other healthcare professionals (Saad, 2022). Thus, nurses are well positioned to navigate frequent ethical dilemmas due to the increasing complexities of the healthcare system.

Developing their knowledge in all areas of care, especially in identifying and resolving ethical dilemmas, is timely and prudent. Ethically sound clinical judgment and competence begins with the graduate curriculum for the more than 234,000 licensed APRNs in the US (American Association of Nurse Practitioners, 2017). The authors discovered that graduating DNP students could not always identify an ethical dilemma (Vermeesch et al., 2019).

APRN students in their clinical rotations appear better prepared to identify ethically challenging situations than students in their didactic-only portion of their programs, despite previous experience as a registered nurse. Once immersed in clinical experiences, students recognize that not all situations have a clear and singular solution. It is possible that while in the didactic portion of their programs, they have not yet developed the skills necessary to identify and voice concerns regarding ethical dilemmas. Understanding ethical frameworks and the process required for critical decision-making allows for the highest provision of patient care.

Determining the appropriate place in APRN programs to introduce and discuss ethical dilemmas is vital in developing effective and relevant APRN curricula. Providing case studies that demonstrate the complexity inherent in caring for humans allows students to broaden their viewpoint and become more aware of potential ethical dilemmas, all while still in their didactic courses; this will allow for a more robust preparation to address ethical challenges when they enter clinical rotations.

We are excited to provide a book that increases the APRN's knowledge and agility in resolving ethical dilemmas encountered in the clinical setting, healthcare organizations, and academic institutions. Our goals for this book are:

- Provide an educational tool to increase APRN students' abilities to identify ethical concerns and work through them to find a solution.

- Inform and expand current ethical pedagogy for APRN students. Faculty teaching in doctor of nursing practice, master

of science in nursing, and certified nurse anesthetist programs; their students; and practicing APRNs will benefit from
working through the case studies to identify and solve ethical
dilemmas.

- Provide classroom and clinical teaching in the form of case
studies to foster critical thinking, judgment, and the skills
needed to resolve ethical dilemmas. As healthcare increases in
complexity, APRNs will continue to experience ethical conflicts and dilemmas. Providing guidance to APRNs in identifying and resolving ethical dilemmas can increase effective
patient outcomes, and we can continue to be the most honest
and ethical profession now and into the future.

Important Information About This Book

The framework we put forth in this book is the American Public
Health Association Model Curriculum in Ethics and Public Health
(Jennings et al., 2003). This model provides a concise method for
identifying and resolving ethical dilemmas. There is not necessarily a
"right" answer to the dilemmas in each case study. The idea is to pro-
voke thought regarding how one may approach the patient concern
from an ethical, moral, and legal standpoint.

The Framework and How to Use It

Consideration for ethics in advanced nursing practice can be taxing,
regardless of where one is in their career. As an APRN with many responsibilities when caring for patients, applying ethical consideration
to each decision can be a daunting task. Not that every situation needs
an in-depth ethical analysis; however, certain circumstances require
more thought and attention. Applying a framework can help the
APRN by providing a set of criteria for working through an ethical
dilemma. It does not provide an answer to the dilemma, but it helps to
guide the APRN to use critical thinking to come to an ethically sound
decision.

Steps to consider to analyze a dilemma using an ethical framework:

- Identify the problem.

- Assess the factual information.

- Identify the involved parties.

- What is at stake?

- What options are available?

- What process is needed to make a decision?

Identify the problem and associated components

What is the problem, and who is involved? The more complex the case, the more important it is to identify the problem clearly. Therefore, the ethical values and concepts are enunciated to define the problem.

Assess the factual information

Gather all the information about the situation. For example, physical characteristics of a patient might not be as important as other medical history to ethical decision-making. Include details of what is not known and what is needed and how to ascertain it. The validity, type, and source of the information is important as well.

Identify the involved stakeholders

Who and how will those involved in any decisions be affected by the outcome? Will those involved be harmed or benefited? Will there be justification for the consequences? Is there intent to harm or benefit by the decision-maker or is it an expected result? Has the person who would be harmed by the decision participated voluntarily knowing the risks involved? Finally, how do all the facts affect the intended and unintended consequences of the decision?

What is at stake?

Identify the worth of the various components of the issue. Worth includes such categories as physical well-being, autonomy, esteem, and respect for self and others. Faculty may consider providing tailored and appropriate values for the context.

What options are available?

Identify the options for decisions to be made. Options are not always clear-cut in their moral weight. It is important to be reflective and to consider all parts of the dilemma. Consider compromise as an appropriate solution.

What process is needed to make a decision?

Be clear in the steps of the selected process and consequences before taking action. Identify who should be making the decision about the process and what other needed roles should be included.

Source: Jennings et al., 2003.

ANA Code of Ethics

To perform at the highest level of their profession, nurses must conduct themselves in an ethical manner. The American Nurses Association (ANA) Code of Ethics for Nurses provides the obligation, values, duties, and standard for the profession. Importantly, the code does not predetermine how those obligations are met; nurses may meet those obligations individually or support their nurse colleagues in meeting those obligations. The code is intended for all nurses no matter their role in practice or setting (Winland-Brown et al., 2015). The main principles that guide ethical behavior are:

- **Autonomy:** "Rational self-legislation and self-determination that is grounded in informedness, voluntariness, consent, and rationality."

- **Beneficence:** "Benefiting others by preventing harm, removing harmful conditions, or affirmatively acting to benefit another or others, often going beyond what is required by law."

- **Justice:** "A bioethical principle with various types or domains of justice, including distributive, retributive, restorative, transitional, intergenerational, and procedural. Bioethics is chiefly concerned with distributive justice. Distributive justice deals with the equitable distribution of social burdens and benefits society. When this allocation occurs under conditions of scarcity, it raises questions of rationing. The formal principle of justice states that equals shall be treated equally, and unequals unequally, in proportion to their relevant differences."

- **Nonmaleficence:** This principle "specifies that a duty not to inflict harm and balances unavoidable harm with benefits of good achieved."

Keep these principles in mind, as well as the nine provisions of the Code of Ethics for Nurses.

ANA CODE OF ETHICS

Provision 1   The nurse practices with compassion and respect for the inherent dignity, worth, and unique attributes of every person.

Provision 2   The nurse's primary commitment is to the patient, whether an individual, family, group, community, or population.

Provision 3   The nurse promotes, advocates for, and protects the rights, health, and safety of the patient.

Provision 4   The nurse has authority, accountability, and responsibility for nursing practice; makes decisions; and takes action consistent with the obligation to promote health and to provide optimal patient care.

Provision 5   The nurse owes the same duties to self as to others, including the responsibility to promote health and safety, preserve wholeness of character and integrity, maintain competence, and continue personal and professional growth.

Provision 6   The nurse, through individual and collective effort, establishes, maintains, and improves the ethical environment of the work setting and conditions of employment that are conducive to safe, quality health care.

Provision 7   The nurse, in all roles and settings, advances the profession through research and scholarly inquiry, professional standards development, and the generation of both nursing and health policy.

Provision 8   The nurse collaborates with other health professionals and the public to protect human rights, promote health diplomacy, and reduce health disparities.

Provision 9   The profession of nursing, collectively through its professional organizations, must articulate nursing values, maintain the integrity of the profession, and integrate principles of social justice into nursing and health policy.

Source: American Nurses Association, 2015.

Terminology

Most nurses have had ethics in their curriculum at the undergraduate level, but a refresher of the terms here will put everyone on an equal footing.

Accountability: Accepting responsibility for one's own actions, including professional and personal consequences that can occur as the result of one's actions.

Advanced practice registered nurse (APRN): A nurse who has the ability to treat and diagnose illnesses, advise the public on health issues, manage chronic disease, and engage in continuous education to remain ahead of any technological, methodological, or other developments in the field. APRNs hold at least a master's degree, in addition to the initial nursing education and licensing required for all registered nurses.

Examples of APRNs:

- Nurse practitioners

- Certified nurse-midwives

- Clinical nurse specialists

- Certified registered nurse anesthetists

Affect: An outward expression of a person's emotional state.

Autonomy: Patient self-determination; the innate right of a person to their own opinions, perspectives, values, and beliefs. Healthcare providers have an obligation to encourage patients to make their own decision without any judgments or coercion.

Bias: Prejudice in favor of or against one thing, person, or group compared with another, usually in a way considered to be unfair.

Case-based learning: It is well documented that case studies are an effective teaching strategy for APRNs as well as other clinicians. They are most useful for providing complex real-world patient situations with multiple layers that can be unfolded and walked through with a clinical expert.

Case study pedagogy: Use of case studies to analyze a dilemma.

Doctor of nursing practice (DNP): The DNP is designed for nurses seeking a terminal degree in nursing practice and offers an alternative to research-focused doctoral programs. DNP-prepared nurses are well equipped to fully implement the science developed by nurse researchers prepared in doctor of philosophy (PhD), doctor of nursing science (DNS), and other research-focused nursing doctorates.

In many institutions, advanced practice registered nurses (APRNs), including nurse practitioner (NP), clinical nurse specialist (CNS), certified nurse midwife (CNM), and certified registered nurse anesthetist (CRNA), are prepared in master's degree programs that often carry a credit load equivalent to doctoral degrees in the other health professions. A position statement from the American Association of Colleges of Nursing (AACN) calls for educating APRNs and other nurses seeking top leadership/organizational roles in DNP programs (AACN, 2004).

There are multiple types of DNP specialties including executive leadership, technology, public health, health policy, and clinically focused specialties: CNM, CRNA, CNS, psychiatric mental health nurse practitioner (PMHNP), neonatal nurse practitioner (NNP), adult gerontology primary care nurse practitioner (AGPCNP), adult gerontology acute care nurse practitioner (AGACNP), pediatric nurse practitioner (PNP), women's health nurse practitioner (WHNP), and family nurse practitioner (FNP). DNP curricula build on traditional master's programs by providing education in evidence-based practice, quality improvement, and systems leadership, among other key areas. The DNP in executive leadership is designed to prepare nurses to lead teams, work at the highest level of advanced practice, and lead in a wide range of healthcare and education organizations.

Ethics: A set of moral principles and patterns of choice that guide behavior.

Fairness: Marked by impartiality and honesty; free from self-interest, prejudice, or favoritism.

Fidelity: Keeping one's promises. Being faithful and true to professional promises and responsibilities by providing high-quality, safe care in a competent manner.

Integrity: Wholeness in the quality of being honest and morally upright.

Long-acting injectable medication: Long-acting injectable formulation of antipsychotic medications can be given typically every two to four weeks, depending on the medication. This medication formulation improves adherence, as individuals do not have to remember to take the medication daily or multiple times a day.

Morals: Principles that guide the understanding of right and wrong.

Principle: A fundamental truth or proposition that serves as the foundation for a system of belief or behavior or for a chain of reasoning.

Values: A set of standards that influence behavior. Examples of values include honesty, integrity, fairness, and concern and respect for others.

Veracity: Being completely truthful; not withholding the whole truth even when it may lead to patient distress.

Final Note

We hope this book empowers APRNs with the critical knowledge and skills to handle even the most complex ethical dilemmas in their practice.

References

American Association of Colleges of Nursing. (2004). *AACN position statement on the practice doctorate in nursing.* https://www.aacnnursing.org/DNP/Position-Statement

American Association of Nurse Practitioners. (2018, August 8). 2017 National Nurse Practitioner Sample Survey results. *AANP News.* https://www.aanp.org/news-feed/2017-national-nurse-practitioner-sample-survey-results

American Nurses Association. (2015). *Code of Ethics for Nurses With Interpretative Statements.* http://www.nursingworld.org/MainMenuCategories/EthicsStandards/CodeofEthicsforNurses/Code-of-Ethics-For-Nurses.html

Community Catalyst. (n.d.). *Primary care: Expanding the use of nurse practitioners.* https://www.communitycatalyst.org/resources/tools/medicaid-report-card/primary-care/primary-care-expanding-the-use-of-nurse-practitioners

HHS.gov. (2021, June 5). *New HHS data show more Americans than ever have health coverage through the Affordable Care Act.* https://www.hhs.gov/about/news/2021/06/05/new-hhs-data-show-more-americans-than-ever-have-health-coverage-through-affordable-care-act.html

Jennings, B., Kahn, J., Mastroianni, A., & Parker, L. S. (2003). *Ethics and public health: Model curriculum.* Association of Schools of Public Health. https://courses.washington.edu/bethics/violations/ASPHEthicsCurriculum.pdf

Levey, N. N. (2021, May 4). A primary care physician for every American, science panel urges. *Kaiser Health News.* https://khn.org/news/article/primary-care-physician-for-every-american-national-academies-recommendation-empanelment/

Saad, L. (2022, January 12). Military brass, judges among professions at new image lows. *Gallup.* https://news.gallup.com/poll/388649/military-brass-judges-among-professions-new-image-lows.aspx

Schiff, M. (2012, December). *The role of nurse practitioners in meeting increasing demand for primary care.* National Governors Association. https://www.nga.org/wp-content/uploads/2019/08/1212NursePractitionersPaper.pdf

Vermeesch, A., Cox, P., Baca, S., & Simmons, D. (2019). Strategies for strengthening ethics education in a DNP program. *Nursing Education Perspectives, 39*(5), 309–311. https://doi.org/10.1097/01.NEP.0000000000000383

Winland-Brown, J., Lachman, V. D., & Swanson, E. O. C. (2015). The new 'Code of Ethics for Nurses With Interpretive Statements' (2015): Practical clinical application, Part I. *Medsurg Nursing, 24*(4), 268–271.

DEFENSIVE MEDICINE

Defensive medicine is a concept first defined in the early 1970s as a medical practice performed by clinicians who have authority to order testing and prescribe medications to patients and do so to reduce the possibility of litigation, regardless of cost or risk of harm (Ünal & Akbolat, 2021). Regrettably, when practicing medicine defensively, the clinician is not thinking about the benefit to the patient and is typically not using modalities for treatment considered to be evidence-based practice (Bester, 2020). Since the initial definition, subsequent definitions have attempted to make the idea of defensive medicine more appealing, such as the "fear of overlooking important findings" or "the willingness to avoid wrongful diagnoses" (Ünal & Akbolat, 2021, para. 1). Still, it is the act of protecting oneself as a medical provider from being sued rather than doing what is best for the patient and cost-effective for the medical system (Bester, 2020).

As controversial as this sounds to put one's career and license before patient care and safety, malpractice is something most healthcare clinicians with ordering and prescriptive authority are acutely aware of and why the practice of defensive medicine may be so prevalent. Malpractice lawsuits near 200,000 cases each year in the United States, equating to approximately 20 billion dollars in paid claims (Feldstein, 2018). The most common paid claims for malpractice suits are for diagnosis errors (31.8%) and medication and treatment errors (24.5%), which affect clinicians in any medical setting (Feldstein, 2018). Not to mention the time, stress, and lost wages a clinician must endure if brought to trial (Feldstein, 2018).

Defensive Medicine: An Ethical Dilemma Case Study

You are a family nurse practitioner working per diem for a family medicine clinic affiliated with a large hospital system in Indianapolis, Indiana. It is the middle of January, and your colleagues have been overwhelmed by the number of ill people coming into the clinic; some are seeing upwards of 27 patients a day. Last year, your clinic took care of a patient who presented with a fever and respiratory symptoms at the time of visit; the patient ended up in the hospital for a month and on a ventilator. The patient's family describes it as a missed/delayed influenza and pneumonia diagnosis. The patient suffered permanent brain damage, and now the family and the attending provider are in the middle of litigation. It is your first day back in the clinic since before the new year, and it is evident from conversations with your colleagues everyone is upset and worried about the recent accusations and lawsuit. Because of the volume of patients seen and for fear of litigation, you have a colleague who began ordering influenza testing via nasopharyngeal swab and a chest X-ray for anyone with a cough or slightest fever. She has also decided to prescribe Tamiflu for anyone with a fever over 102, regardless of the result of the influenza swab. The first patient on your schedule is a 44-year-old African American woman, Eva, and her appointment note reads "Flu-Like Symptoms." After the patient has checked in and is ready to go, you review your medical assistant's note and vital signs to discover Eva's chief complaint is fatigue, a productive cough, and a terrible headache for almost two days. You put on proper personal protective equipment and enter the room.

As you discuss the course of illness thus far with Eva, you find she has no known exposers, her symptoms came on gradually over a day, and Tylenol is helping to bring her fever down and decrease symptoms of myalgia. She states she has "the worst headache" that began quickly after she started feeling ill; this seems to be bothering her most. Upon physical exam, Eva looks ill but is not in acute distress. Blood pressure is 126/68, pulse 82, temperature 101.6, respiration 15, and oxygen saturation is 98%. She is found to have slight bronchial wheezing in bilateral upper chest, productive sounding cough, moderate nasal congestion, and cervical lymphadenopathy. The rest of her physical exam is within normal limits. You believe the diagnosis to be an acute upper respiratory infection. Still, against your better judgment, knowledge, and experience, you find yourself torn. Should you do a chest X-ray just in case? And knowing that influenza is prevalent, should you test for that as well? The headache seemed to be bothering Eva and had an abrupt onset; she also said it was "the worst," so you consider a computed tomography (CT) scan. All these things seem unnecessary to you, but could it prevent a lawsuit if this patient does have something more severe than just a common cold?

How may you go about managing this situation so you are able to care for Eva and keep yourself safe from possible litigation?

Consider:

1. Identify the ethical concerns with this situation.

2. What information will you need before a responsible decision can be made? (Consider what the information is and where it will come from.)

3. Who are stakeholders involved in the decision, and what is the process in which those involved could come to a decision (e.g., what tools are/could be used to create an informed decision)?

4. What are the values relevant to this problem? *Values* are the things that you believe are important in making the decision. They (should) determine priorities. Values relevant to this problem may not be representative of your own personal values or moral framework.

5. What are the options for the decision? Think in terms of values and feasibility (e.g., financial, political, organizational, religious constraints).

Management of Case Study

After all considerations, write a short narrative of how you believe is the best way to manage this situation; list core values important to you for managing the situation.

References

Bester, J. C. (2020). Defensive practice is indefensible: How defensive medicine runs counter to the ethical and professional obligations of clinicians. *Medicine, Health Care and Philosophy, 23*(3), 413–420. https://doi.org/10.1007/s11019-020-09950-7

Feldstein, P. (2018). *Health policy issues: An economic perspective* (7th ed.). Health Administration Press.

Ünal, Ö., & Akbolat, M. (2021). Defensive medicine practices: Scale development and validation. *Medical Decision Making, 42*(2), 255–261. https://doi.org/10.1177/0272989x211043077

STI CONFIDENTIALITY

Confidentiality is fundamental to the nursing profession. Nurses have sworn to this ethical code as far back as 1893 when Lystra E. Gretter composed the Florence Nightingale pledge, which states, "I will do all in my power to maintain and elevate the standard of my profession and will hold in confidence all personal matters committed to my keeping" (Gilbert, 2020). However, as time has passed and the world has changed, circumstances have been identified when the nurse may need to disclose private information about their patient, especially if the information puts the patient or someone else at risk of harm (Centers for Disease Control, 2021). For example, patients often present to their nurse practitioner (NP) at their family medicine clinic, urgent care, or the hospital seeking care that requires screening and/or treatment for a sexually transmitted infection (STI). Unfortunately, an STI found in an individual patient is not the only concern for the NP. It is well documented that these infections are mainly transmitted through direct sexual contact, and not all people who have an STI become symptomatic right away, if at all. Thus, if someone screens positive for an STI, all partners having recent sexual contact with the infected person must be screened and treated as well to lessen spread. However, this is easier said than done. Historically, there has been shame and stigma surrounding STIs. As a result, those who suspect they have an STI are often unwilling to be tested until they become severely symptomatic, and if found to be positive, they are ashamed and reluctant to tell their partners, even though keeping that information from their partners may be detrimental (Laar, DeBruin, & Craddock, 2015). Consequently, the concept of mandatory reporting of STIs to public health departments became a topic of debate. In the 1990s, when HIV and AIDS had reached epidemic proportions, Gostin and Hodge (1998, p. 11) profoundly stated, "Secrecy nurtures disease by providing an environment conducive to the spread of infection." They discuss how the earliest and most effective recorded public health strategy for STI prevention was the introduction of the "duty to warn," which mandates provider reporting and health department notification for sexual partners of infected patients.

Many state legislatures require healthcare providers to report positive STI results to county health departments. Several states also require partner identification if they are known. Partner identification allows county health departments to confidentially notify potential positive cases, which aids in mitigating the spread of STI infection in the community.

STI Confidentiality Case Study

You are a family nurse practitioner working in Austin, Texas, at an outpatient family practice clinic. Today is Monday, and as you look over your schedule, you find your day filled with several typical appointment types, such as chronic care management, complete physicals, acute illnesses and injury, etc. You notice Amy, a 29-year-old married woman and mother of two, is on your schedule. Amy and her entire family are some of the first patients to become a part of your personal patient panel. Thus, you have been caring for Amy for some time now and are aware of her history and current problems. She is a relatively healthy young woman who has been seen for anxiety and depression three times in the last 10 months. Much of these concerns began because of her relationship with her husband. Since having children, her husband has been more distant, inattentive, and easily frustrated with her and their family situation. Amy has relayed that he does not help with the children or the household duties and tends to be absent when things get complicated. However, at her last visit, her depression and anxiety were much more well-controlled after seeing a therapist and starting on a low-dose selective serotonin reuptake inhibitor (SSRI), all of which she is doing without the knowledge or support of her husband. As she has told you, he would think she is "crazy" if he knew she was being treated for a mental health condition. Today her appointment is labeled "confidential," which is odd to you, and as you look back on her historical appointment notes, they have always indicated the reason for her visit. Regardless, you believe it is likely for her anxiety and depression and are looking forward to seeing her in clinic.

Amy arrives on time for her appointment; your medical assistant (MA) brings her back and gets the chief complaint and vital signs. However, as you prepare her chart, you notice the chief complaint states "confidential," and there are no documented vital signs. You find your assigned MA and ask about her interaction with Amy. The MA tells you that Amy began to cry as soon as she brought her back. Amy then declined to have vital signs taken and stated she wanted to talk to you and only you about why she was there for the appointment. You enter the room to find Amy in tears. Giving her a tissue, you ask what happened to make her so upset. Eventually, she calms down and discloses to you she has been having an affair for the last six months with a younger man. She goes on to tell you that she has had unprotected sex multiple times with the young man and received word yesterday after he visited an urgent care clinic he tested positive for gonorrhea. Amy has continued to have unprotected intercourse with her husband as well. She imparts that she really did not want to but thought he would have gotten upset and become suspicious if she did not. She is on birth control pills and takes them daily; thus, she does not think she is pregnant.

On review of systems, you note she does not have any severe symptoms; however, she has had mild intermittent lower abdominal pain and some burning with urination for the last month. Initially, she thought the symptoms were from a mild urinary tract infection and has been hydrating well and drinking cranberry juice, with no real improvement of symptoms. She denies urgency, frequency, or hematuria. She also notes that she has had an increase in vaginal discharge and a bit of spotting between her periods, even though she has been on birth control over the last few months.

On gynecologic exam, you note a moderate amount of thin, white, slightly odorous discharge and mild cervical motion tenderness. No adnexal tenderness. Because you are doing a vaginal exam, you take cultures for gonorrhea and chlamydia.

Amy likely has gonorrhea as she has had significant exposure and is symptomatic. Unless she is treated, it is possible to develop more severe and long-term complications from the infection. It is also important that any partner she has had be treated as well, so they do not develop complications; this includes her husband. As you are discussing the treatment for gonorrhea, you advise her that it is one intramuscular injection and one oral medication that can be done in the office for both her and her husband. She begins to cry again and says she cannot tell her husband and begs you not to tell him either. You then advise her that even if neither of you tell her husband, you are required by Texas law to report all STI cases and known partners to the county health department (Texas Department of State Health Services, n.d.). They will likely contact him to let him know he may have been ex- posed. She begins to panic and blurts out, "But he's gonna beat me if he finds out." She continues to beg you not to notify the county and tells you that if you just give her the medication, she will make sure she and her husband get it. You were unaware of any physical violence in the home, and you begin to wonder how you will handle this with the least amount of harm coming to all parties involved.

With the information that Amy likely has a reportable STI, Texas law, how the medications for gonorrhea must be given, and the panicked nature of the patient out of fear for her safety, how might you legally and ethically approach this situation?

Consider:

1. Identify the ethical concerns with this situation.

2. What information will you need before a responsible decision can be made? (Consider what the information is and where it will come from.)

3. Who are stakeholders involved in the decision, and what is the process in which those involved could come to a decision (e.g., what tools are/could be used to create an informed decision)?

4. What are the values relevant to this problem? *Values* are the things that you believe are important in making the decision. They (should) determine priorities. Values relevant to this problem may not be representative of your own personal values or moral framework.

5. What are the options for the decision? Think in terms of values and feasibility (e.g., financial, political, organizational, religious constraints).

Management of Case Study

After all considerations, write a short narrative of how you believe is the best way to manage this situation; list core values important to you for managing the situation.

References

Centers for Disease Control and Prevention. (2021, May 3). *Duty to warn.* https://www.cdc.gov/std/treatment/duty-to-warn.htm

Gilbert, H. A. (2020). Florence Nightingale's environmental theory and its influence on contemporary infection control. *Collegian, 27*(6), 626–633.

Gostin, L. O., & Hodge, J. G. (1998). Piercing the veil of secrecy in HIV/AIDS and other sexually transmitted diseases: Theories of privacy and disclosure in partner notification. *Duke Journal of Gender Law & Policy, 5*(1), 9–88.

Laar, A. K., DeBruin, D. A., & Craddock, S. (2015). Partner notification in the context of HIV: An interest-analysis. *AIDS Research and Therapy, 12*(1). https://doi.org/10.1186/s12981-015-0057-8

Texas Department of State Health Services. (n.d.). *HIV/STI partner services and seropositive notification.* https://www.dshs.texas.gov/hivstd/pops/chap03.shtm

CASE STUDY #3

SUBSTANCE USE IN PREGNANCY

The opioid health crisis continues to be an uphill battle in the US. When it comes to pregnant women and their unborn infants, provider concern for those involved is centered not only on the person using opioids but also on the fetus (Ecker et al., 2019). Other considerations include stigma and shame projected by the public and healthcare providers for pregnant women identified with or treated for a substance use disorder (Ecker et al., 2019). Often, they find themselves labeled as child abusers, and their rights as parents are contested or taken away (Ecker et al., 2019).

Yet, there is mounting evidence that substance use disorder is a disease, "not a moral failing," and should be treated as such, even in the setting of a pregnant woman (Ecker et al., 2019, p. B22). However, legally in the US, 18 states define substance use in pregnancy as child abuse, and three states consider it grounds for jail time (Ecker et al., 2019). Thus, these women can be arrested, prosecuted, and/or incarcerated for drug use (Ecker et al., 2019).

According to Ecker et al. (2019), several medical and ethical issues should be considered when a woman is using and there is an unborn child involved. Focused discussions and considerations should include the woman's autonomy when undergoing screening or treatment, truth when discussing plans for treatment and care, justice to ensure care available to every other pregnant woman is available to her, and nonmaleficence and beneficence, for both mother and baby (Ecker et al., 2019).

Substance Use in Pregnancy Case Study

You are a nurse-midwife working in a women's health clinic in West Virginia. Your day is busy seeing pregnant and postpartum women, as well as women with other gynecological health concerns. Currently, you are preparing to see 36-year-old Melissa. She has not been seen in your clinic before and comes in today to seek care for her current pregnancy and discuss symptoms of a urinary tract infection (UTI). Your medical assistant (MA) brings her back and confirms her pregnancy with a human chorionic gonadotropin urine test and the presence of a UTI with a urine dip. The MA also attempts to establish her last menstrual period and pregnancy history, which is difficult because of the patient's lack of accurate recall. Your MA gives you the information she was able to gather, and before you enter the patient's room, you calculate current gestation based on her last menstrual period, and you believe her to be at 18–20 weeks gestation. You also establish that she is a Gravida 3 Para 0 (G3P0), with one spontaneous and one induced abortion and now this current pregnancy. Your MA advises that the patient had seen her general practitioner early on and was told she was at too high risk of continuing her pregnancy and should consider abortion. Hence, she decided not to seek care again until now.

The patient continued by saying that the only reason she was seeking care now was because she was able to find a nurse and not a physician, and she thinks she may have an infection. You enter the room to find a tall, very thin Caucasian woman with long wavy hair and several tattoos. Her eyes and cheeks appear sunken, and she has sores at various stages of healing on her face and arms. After greeting her, you introduce yourself. You come to find that Melissa uses methamphet-amine via intravenous (IV) injection. However, since learning about the pregnancy, she has been using much less than before the pregnan-cy. She tells you, "I've been trying to cut back and even stop for the baby, but I can't stop; my friend told me I could die if I just stop." You discuss treatment for the UTI and what she would need to do moving forward with the pregnancy to ensure her baby is safe. You tell her that she and her baby are at higher risk for complications because of the IV drug use; however, you can help her get the care she and her baby need if she is willing. Melissa says, "I don't trust those doctors. If you're gonna send me to a doctor, I ain't gonna go."

Consider

1. Identify the ethical concerns with this situation.

2. What information will you need before a responsible decision can be made? (Consider what the information is and where it will come from.)

3. Who are stakeholders involved in the decision, and what is the process in which those involved could come to a deci-sion (e.g., what tools are/could be used to create an informed decision)?

4. What are the values relevant to this problem? *Values* are the things that you believe are important in making the decision. They (should) determine priorities. Values relevant to this problem may not be representative of your own personal values or moral framework.

5. What are the options for the decision? Think in terms of values and feasibility (e.g., financial, political, organizational, religious constraints).

Management of Case Study

After all considerations, write a short narrative of how you believe is the best way to manage this situation; list core values important to you for managing the situation.

Reference

Ecker, J., Abuhamad, A., Hill, W., Bailit, J., Bateman, B. T., Berghella, V., Blake-Lamb, T., Guille, C., Landau, R., Minkoff, H., Prabhu, M., Rosenthal, E., Terplan, M., Wright, T. E., & Yonkers, K. A. (2019). Substance use disorders in pregnancy: Clinical, ethical, and research imperatives of the opioid epidemic: A report of a joint workshop of the Society for Maternal-Fetal Medicine, American College of Obstetricians and Gynecologists, and American Society of Addiction Medicine. *American Journal of Obstetrics and Gynecology, 221*(1), B5–B28. https://doi.org/10.1016/j.ajog.2019.03.022

HPV VACCINE REFUSAL

The human papillomavirus (HPV) is a viral infection passed from person to person through skin-to-skin contact (Centers for Disease Control and Prevention [CDC], 2022). There are many types of HPV, many of which are contracted via sexual contact (CDC, 2022). The CDC (2022) notes that HPV is the most common sexually transmitted disease in the United States. Most people will get some form of HPV in their lifetime if they become sexually active, regardless of the number of sexual partners (CDC, 2022). HPV is also the leading cause of cervical cancer in the United States, even though there is a vaccine that is proven effective against the cancer-causing high-risk variants such as HPV 16 and 18 (CDC, 2022).

The human papillomavirus vaccine (2vHPV, 4vHPV, 9vHPV) was first introduced in the US in 2006 (VanWormer et al., 2017). At that time, the vaccine was intended to be given to adolescent girls aged 11–12 to protect them from future cervical cancer. It is now recommended for both adolescent boys and girls aged 9–14 to receive the vaccine. The HPV vaccine has been shown to reduce the risk of cervical infection with high-risk HPV by over 90% (Sundaram et al., 2019). Vaccinating all genders allow for the protection of both the individual and their future sexual partners. However, a small portion of the adolescent population becomes vaccinated against HPV compared to other adolescent vaccinations such as the tetanus, diphtheria, and pertussis (Tdap) vaccine, and the vaccine to protect from meningococcal disease (MCV4). HPV vaccine completion is estimated at only 35% in the US (VanWormer et al., 2017). The explanations for low vaccination rates have not been well researched; however, several reasons are thought to be related to parental hesitancies, ambivalence, or resistance when deciding on vaccinating their children against HPV (VanWormer et al., 2017). These include the adolescent's young age and their presumed timeline until sexual exposure and parents' underestimation of their child's susceptibility to acquiring STIs or cervical cancer (VanWormer et al., 2017). Parents also tend to focus on and overemphasize the risks of the HPV vaccine, such as adverse reactions (VanWormer et al., 2017). Unfortunately, some of the reactions are realistic and short term such as syncope immediately following vaccination; however, others were at one time speculated and proven to be false claims, such as thromboembolism and risky sexual behaviors (VanWormer et al., 2017).

There are distinctions with the HPV vaccine that differentiate it from other childhood vaccinations. One, the vaccine is intended to be given in adolescence, so protection from the virus is well established prior to exposure, which may be well beyond adolescent years (VanWormer et al., 2017). There are also other ways to protect against the virus, such as not participating in sexual activities and using safe sex practices to prevent HPV (VanWormer et al., 2017). It is also known with HPV that female health is disproportionately affected by the virus due to the risk of HPV developing into cervical cancer (VanWormer et al., 2017). Thus, not all insurance carriers will cover the HPV vaccine for males; however, as more data are becoming available on the benefit of vaccinating males against HPV, this is becoming less of a concern. These differences may affect parents' and patients' decisions on vaccination at the recommended age.

It is important to note that although HPV affects the female gender at a higher rate than males, boys and men are not innately immune to the consequences of HPV infection, especially in men who participate in sex with other men. Men tend to have a higher risk of developing oral HPV infections and a higher risk of specific cancers, such as head and neck cancers, as a result.

HPV Vaccine Case Study

You are a family nurse practitioner working for a busy practice in Seattle, Washington. You are going over your schedule with the medical assistant (MA) and see that 14-year-old Ethan is on your schedule for a routine well-child exam/sports physical. You have been taking care of Ethan since he was an infant; however, it has been several years since you have seen him. You look up his vaccination history on the state registry, and he is a bit behind. Ethan has not had his 11-12-year-old series, consisting of the Tdap, MCV4, and HPV. His mother Rhonda comes to all his appointments and is pro-vaccination to your recollection and historical chart notes. Thus, you prepare the MA to give the Vaccine Information Statement forms for Ethan's vaccines. When Ethan is checked in, the MA advises you that Rhonda has agreed for Ethan to receive the Tdap and MCV4; however, she has declined the HPV vaccine. The MA left the HPV vaccine information sheet in the room for Rhonda and advised her to discuss questions and concerns about the vaccine with you.

After entering the room, you perform a history and physical examination to find everything within normal limits for his age and development. You ask Ethan's mother to leave the room so you can discuss a few more personal things with him; Rhonda respectfully leaves the room. You discuss several things, such as body image, self-esteem, reproduction, and sexual activity. Ethan reports he is content with himself and is not sexually active; however, he likes a girl at school more than a friend. Ethan admits to you they have been affectionate at times by kissing and holding hands, but nothing beyond that. You ask Ethan how he feels about getting his vaccinations, including the HPV vaccine, and he reveals he doesn't care if he gets his vaccines and states, "It's up to my mom."

Overall, you assess Ethan as a young, healthy adolescent boy. When his mother reenters the room, you discuss your findings, as well as the vaccinations Ethan is due for. Rhonda again relays she does not want Ethan to receive the HPV vaccine. You ask her about her concerns regarding the vaccine. Rhonda communicates she worries the vaccine may allow children to be more sexually promiscuous. Beyond this, she states, "Plus, I'm not worried about Ethan getting HPV; he's a boy." She also discusses how she has heard about fainting and death resulting from the vaccine, so it doesn't make sense to her to vaccinate Ethan when there is a risk for adverse events and no risk he will get the disease.

With your knowledge of the HPV vaccine, how would/could you respond to Rhonda's concerns about the HPV vaccine?

Consider:

1. Identify the ethical concerns with this situation.

2. What information will you need before a responsible decision can be made? (Consider what the information is and where it will come from.)

3. Who are stakeholders involved in the decision, and what is the process in which those involved could come to a decision (e.g., what tools are/could be used to create an informed decision)?

4. What are the values relevant to this problem? *Values* are the things that you believe are important in making the decision. They (should) determine priorities. Values relevant to this problem may not be representative of your own personal values or moral framework.

5. What are the options for the decision? Think in terms of values and feasibility (e.g., financial, political, organizational, religious constraints).

Management of Case Study

After all considerations, write a short narrative of how you believe is the best way to manage this situation; list core values important to you for managing the situation.

4

References

Centers for Disease Control and Prevention. (2022, January 20). *HPV fact sheet.* https://www.cdc.gov/std/hpv/stdfact-hpv.htm

Sundaram, N., Voo, T. C., & Tam, C. C. (2019). Adolescent HPV vaccination: Empowerment, equity and ethics. *Human Vaccines & Immunotherapeutics, 16*(8), 1835–1840. https://doi.org/10.1080/21645515.2019.1697596

VanWormer, J. J., Bendixsen, C. G., Vickers, E. R., Stokley, S., McNeil, M. M., Gee, J., Belongia, E. A., & McLean, H. Q. (2017). Association between parent attitudes and receipt of human papillomavirus vaccine in adolescents. *BMC Public Health, 17*(1). https://doi.org/10.1186/s12889-017-4787-5

ABORTION

Some consider access to safe abortion a fundamental human right (Mainey et al., 2020). According to Erdman et al. (2013), having access to this type of family planning care has influenced a substantial decline in maternal mortality and morbidity, not only in the developed world but worldwide. Regardless of the established benefit and proof of lifesaving effectiveness, women must continue to seek unsafe abortions because of restrictions and lack of access to safe and legal options (Mainey et al., 2020). Even in developed countries, such as the United States, approximately 30 women of every 100,000 will die from complications related to unsafe abortions (Mainey et al., 2020). The past has shown us that law does not keep a woman from taking matters into her own hands, and she will find a way to terminate an undesired pregnancy, regardless of risk, if her reproductive rights are taken from her (Berer, 2017). However, some healthcare providers continue to find themselves at odds with caring for patients requesting abortion services, especially when it conflicts with law or their religion, morals, or ethical values. When this occurs, the question becomes how the provider can find a way to protect the law and their morals while serving the patient and providing care that will result in the least amount of harm possible (Buchbinder et al., 2016).

On June 24, 2022, the US Supreme Court ruled to overturn Roe vs. Wade's historic 1973 trial decision, which constitutionally protected abortion rights. Today, federal protection of abortion rights does not exist, and it is up to each state to decide whether to allow women to seek abortion care or for health professionals to offer reproductive care of this kind (Robert, 2022). Some states have made "trigger" laws that ban abortion entirely at any stage of gestational development, including cases of incest and rape (Robert, 2022). Violators of these laws, both women and healthcare providers, can face criminal charges, including up to 10 years in prison and significant fines of up to $100,000 (Robert, 2022). At the time of this writing, all states make exceptions if a pregnancy presents life-threatening complications to the woman.

Even after Roe vs. Wade's overturn, many states still continue to allow abortion care for women. States on the West Coast, such as Oregon, and the East Coast, such as New York, have regulations that protect abortion rights and the practitioners that provide abortion care—exceptions to performing an abortion procedure in these states being a viable fetus (Center for Reproductive Rights, n.d.).

Abortion Case Study

You have been working as a family nurse practitioner (FNP) for the better part of two decades. Recently you moved to rural Oregon from Boise, Idaho, to be closer to your family. Family is of utmost priority to you as you are a devoted wife and mother to three grown children and five grandchildren. You and your family have been baptized as part of the Christian faith and attend church regularly. About a month ago, you began working for the largest primary care facility in the area and are mainly seeing overflow patients from your colleagues as you are still building your patient panel. Today, Mariah, a 19-year-old girl you have not met, is on your schedule. Her appointment note states, "needs birth control." You believe this will be a reasonably straightforward appointment as you are well up-to-date with women's reproductive health and have prescribed birth control for patients your entire career as an FNP.

Before you see the patient, you gather your contraception patient information sheet and toolbox so that you can show her all the different options she has to choose from for birth control. As you enter the room to see Mariah, you set your things down, say hello, and introduce yourself. Mariah tells you she just started college in hopes of one day becoming a nurse. You congratulate her and begin to discuss birth control options when she becomes very quiet and starts to seem a bit uncomfortable. You stop and ask if she is OK and if you are going too fast for her. She says, "No, it's fine, but I think I may already be pregnant. Will any of these things help get rid of it if I am?" You stop as you realize that birth control may not be what the patient needs. You ask her why she believes she may be pregnant, and Mariah says she has not had a period in almost eight weeks, and her period is usually right on time; however, she has not taken a pregnancy test. She has also been tired, nauseous, and her breasts have been mildly tender the last few weeks. Mariah goes on to tell you that she had unprotected sex with a guy that she met at a college party about a month and a half ago. You confirm with her that the interaction was consensual and then send her to the clinic lab for a pregnancy test, asking her to return to the room when she is done leaving a urine sample. You move on to see another patient while you are awaiting the results.

In your mind, you are contemplating how you will manage the situation if she is pregnant and what her expectations are. You have run into situations like this in the past; however, all the women were older and eventually decided to continue their pregnancy. Ten minutes pass, and you receive confirmation that Mariah is pregnant. You reenter the room and let her know, and she begins to cry and says, "How could this happen to me? I have to get rid of it. Can you help me get rid of it? Please, you have to; if you don't, I will have to quit college, I will never become a nurse, and my life will be over." You continue to discuss Mariah's options with her, and she tells you, "I know what I have to do if I want to have a future." She goes on to say she has thought about it for the last week, and if she were to find out she was pregnant today, she would discuss options for termination. You know that in Oregon, you can prescribe medication to help terminate a pregnancy before 10 weeks. However, as a Christian, you do not believe in abortion and feel it is a sin to provide care that would result in the termination of a pregnancy. You could refer her to someone else; however, there are no local resources available, and she tells you she does not currently have transportation to a more urban area that does.

Knowing that time is an issue, considering the needs of the patient and your moral values, how might you move forward in caring for this patient?

Consider:

1. Identify the ethical concerns with this situation.

2. What information will you need before a responsible decision can be made? (Consider what the information is and where it will come from.)

3. Who are stakeholders involved in the decision, and what is the process in which those involved could come to a decision (e.g., what tools are/could be used to create an informed decision)?

4. What are the values relevant to this problem? *Values* are the things that you believe are important in making the decision. They (should) determine priorities. Values relevant to this problem may not be representative of your own personal values or moral framework.

5. What are the options for the decision? Think in terms of values and feasibility (e.g., financial, political, organizational, religious constraints).

Management of Case Study

After all considerations, write a short narrative of how you believe is the best way to manage this situation; list core values important to you for managing the situation.

References

Berer, M. (2017). Abortion law and policy around the world: In search of decriminalization. *Health and Human Rights, 19*(1), 13–27. https://europepmc.org/articles/PMC5473035?pdf=render

Buchbinder, M., Lassiter, D., Mercier, R., Bryant, A., & Lyerly, A. D. (2016). Reframing conscientious care: Providing abortion care when law and conscience collide. *Hastings Center Report, 46*(2), 22–30. https://doi.org/10.1002/hast.545

Center for Reproductive Rights. (n.d.). *After Roe fell: Abortion laws by state.* https://reproductiverights.org/maps/abortion-laws-by-state/

Erdman, J. N., DePiñeres, T., & Kismödi, E. (2013). Updated WHO guidance on safe abortion: Health and human rights. *International Journal of Gynecology & Obstetrics, 120*(2), 200–203. https://doi.org/10.1016/j.ijgo.2012.10.009

Hughes, B. (2021). *87(R) SB 8 - House Committee Report version* [PDF]. Texas Legislature online. https://capitol.texas.gov/tlodocs/87R/billtext/pdf/SB00008H.pdf

Mainey, L., O'Mullan, C., Reid-Searl, K., Taylor, A., & Baird, K. (2020). The role of nurses and midwives in the provision of abortion care: A scoping review. *Journal of Clinical Nursing, 29*(9-10), 1513–1526. https://doi.org/10.1111/jocn.15218

Robert, A. (2022). What are abortion trigger laws, and where do they stand? *ABA Journal.* https://www.abajournal.com/web/article/what-are-abortion-trigger-laws-and-where-do-they-stand

PROSTATE CANCER SCREENING WITH PROSTATE-SPECIFIC ANTIGEN

The Food and Drug Administration approved testing for prostate cancer screening in 1994 (Qureshi et al., 2015). Today, almost three decades have passed since the prostate-specific antigen (PSA) was first used as a screening tool in men, with the hopes of detecting early prostate cancer if it is present (Qureshi et al., 2015). Yet over the last decade, recommendations for using the PSA to detect early stages of prostate cancer have changed several times due to the potential lack of accuracy and undue harm that have come to patients attributable to false-positive results. In fact, in 2012, the US Preventive Services Task Force (USPSTF) issued a grade D recommendation, meaning routine PSA screening should not be offered at all (Mishra, 2020). This was because research before 2012 showed prostate cancer screening with PSA resulted in a false-positive screen in up to 80% of men (Qureshi et al., 2015). Most of these men were eventually sent for an unnecessary biopsy of their prostate gland, which can come with substantial unnecessary side effects (Qureshi et al., 2015). However, in 2018 the USPSTF revised its recommendation to grade C, which indicates only to offer PSA testing to men (aged 55–69 years) when shared deci-sion-making is offered (Mishra, 2020). Thus, there are no clear guide-lines, which puts the onus on the provider to discuss risks and benefits and the patient to decide whether they want the screening.

PSA Case Study

You are a geriatric nurse practitioner (GNP) working for a busy family practice in urban Portland, Oregon. The practice consists of you, as the only GNP, and four other providers (three physicians and one physician assistant). You have been working as a GNP for about a year now, your schedule is full, and you are running about 10 minutes be-hind. You enter the room to find a 61-year-old Caucasian man, Steve, in for a routine physical exam. He is a new patient to you, but not the clinic, as he usually sees one of your physician colleagues who is out on vacation. You look through Steve's chart and note that he takes metoprolol 25mg for hypertension, a multivitamin, and an occasional ibuprofen for knee and lower back pain. His vital signs are weight: 179 pounds, height: 71 inches, body mass index: 23.62, blood pres-sure: 122/74, pulse: 61, temperature: 98.4. You discuss Steve's social and family history to discover he is a non-smoker who exercises five days a week and consumes a well-balanced diet, with minimal alcohol intake. Heart disease and diabetes run in Steve's family on his mother's side; he has an older brother who is a smoker, has diabetes, and had a myocardial infarction two years ago. Family history on his father's side includes hypertension and stroke. There is no personal or family history of cancer.

On review of systems, your patient has no concerns; he denies changes to urinary habits and has normal urine flow and output. He does not have symptoms of dribbling at the end of urination or incontinence and denies nocturia. You do your physical assessment, and everything seems to be within normal limits, including the prostate exam. You find the prostate average size and consistency without nodules or masses. Following the physical assessment, you recommend some routine blood tests to screen for high cholesterol, high blood sugar, anemia, and check organ function. You are about to leave the room and walk Steve to the lab when he asks about having his PSA labs done. You advise him that he is at low risk for prostate cancer with his physical exam and social and family history, and there is no indication for routine screening. You begin to educate Steve on why the PSA is no longer routinely done when he stops you and says, "So, last year my doctor said it was very important to have my PSA checked every year; I guess I am just confused about what I should do now." You look at past lab results, and sure enough, there is a PSA result from the year prior that showed a value of 1.2 (with a reference range of less than 4). After discussing his past results and the risks and benefits of PSA screening, he is undecided and would like for you to talk to his PCP before ordering the PSA. As you show Steve out, you let him know you will consult with your colleague and call him with the recommendation following that conversation. After your colleague returns from vacation, you approach him to discuss ordering the PSA for your mutual patient. Your colleague is a male physician who has been practicing for over 20 years. He is not the easiest to talk to, but you know you need to discuss ordering the PSA for Steve. You explain the situation and why you hesitate to recommend the PSA for this patient. He interrupts you and says, "Don't be ridiculous. We have done this for years, and I will not change how I do things for my patients because the government has decided to change its mind on what they will pay to screen for. Besides, it's not going to hurt anyone and will give us information."

After having this conversation, think about how you would proceed with Steve and your colleague.

Consider:

1. Identify the ethical concerns with this situation.

2. What information will you need before a responsible decision can be made? (Consider what the information is and where it will come from.)

3. Who are stakeholders involved in the decision, and what is the process in which those involved could come to a decision (e.g., what tools are/could be used to create an informed decision)?

4. What are the values relevant to this problem? *Values* are the things that you believe are important in making the decision. They (should) determine priorities. Values relevant to this problem may not be representative of your own personal values or moral framework.

5. What are the options for the decision? Think in terms of values and feasibility (e.g., financial, political, organizational, religious constraints).

Management of Case Study

After all considerations, write a short narrative of how you believe is the best way to manage this situation; list core values important to you for managing the situation.

References

Mishra, S. (2020). A discussion on controversies and ethical dilemmas in prostate cancer screening. *Journal of Medical Ethics*, 47(3), 152–158. https://doi.org/10.1136/medethics-2019-105979

Qureshi, Z. P., Bennett, C., Hermanson, T., Horner, R., Haider, R., Lee, M., & Ablin, R. J. (2015). The ethical dilemma surrounding prostate specific antigen (PSA) screening. *Journal of Clinical Research & Bioethics*, 6(1). https://doi.org/10.4172/2155-9627.1000206

ADMINISTRATION OF LONG-ACTING INJECTABLE ANTIPSYCHOTICS

Family nurse practitioners (FNPs) are often the first to learn about a patient's mental illnesses (Balestra, 2019). It is within an FNP's scope to diagnose and treat patients with uncomplicated mental illness, such as depression and anxiety (Balestra, 2019). However, FNPs must know what falls outside of their scope. It is not appropriate for an FNP to diagnose and treat patients with complicated or severe mental illnesses (Balestra, 2019). Any breach of an FNP's scope could lead to disciplinary actions by the board of nursing and could lead to litigation (Balestra, 2019). FNPs should consider and utilize best practices to ensure patient safety and to protect themselves and their license (Balestra, 2019).

Administration of Long-Acting Injectable Antipsychotics Case Study

You are a new-to-practice FNP orienting in a rural community health center with an FNP who is preparing to retire and whose patient panel you will be assuming. Today you are seeing Mark, a 26-year-old Caucasian male with bipolar disorder who was recently released from an acute psychiatric hospitalization. Mark was first diagnosed with major depression by his FNP at age 19 and experienced his first manic episode at age 22 when his diagnosis was updated to bipolar disorder, type one. That manic episode was in the context of starting his first job after graduation from college and involved decreased need for sleep, impulsive spending, and beginning a trip across the country, but coming back home at the behest of his parents. He attended a partial hospitalization program where he was seen by a psychiatrist, participated in group therapy, and was started on olanzapine and maintained on fluoxetine. He had reportedly been doing well for the last four years, working part time and living with his parents.

Mark was recently brought to the local emergency department by the police after running out of his house and down the middle of his busy street. He had become scared that his parents had become possessed. In addition to his psychotic thoughts and disorganized behavior, for three weeks prior, he had been experiencing a decreased need for sleep, with no sleep the two days prior to admission, along with an increased impulse for online shopping (to the point of maxing out his credit card). He had also started to write a novel and had become religiously preoccupied. Before this episode, he had not been interested in writing or religion. He stopped taking his oral olanzapine about four months before his hospitalization because he had gained 20 lbs., become pre-diabetic, and felt "zombie like" most of the time. However, he continued to take his fluoxetine for depression as he feared having another major depressive episode. This was his second manic episode and first hospitalization.

During his admission, Mark was initially reluctant to take medications, he had no behavioral dyscontrol, and he did not require mechanical restraint or seclusion. He began taking oral medications after talking more with psychiatry staff about his concerns regarding medications and learning more about bipolar disorder. He was stabilized on oral aripiprazole. Before discharge, he was given an injection of aripiprazole maintena (a long-acting injectable version of the same medication) and tapered off oral aripiprazole.

Mark is now due for his second injection and presents to the clinic as planned to receive it. There were no mental health providers in the county available to administer the maintena injection for three months, so the FNP agreed to "bridge" him until he could receive care from a prescriber at the community mental health clinic. Before making this decision, the FNP discussed the patient's ongoing care with the inpatient unit's psychiatric mental health nurse practitioner. The FNP would also be responsible for monitoring reemerging symptoms of mania and side effects from the medication, as well as work closely with Mark's parents and community case manager to manage his ongoing needs until his mental health prescriber appointment.

Mark presents as slightly guarded with a linear and organized thought process. He states he is embarrassed about his behavior prior to his hospitalization. His affect is reactive and congruent to mood. He reports he has been sleeping well, averaging eight to nine hours a night, and feeling a little groggy in the morning. He has no overt symptoms of psychosis and is denying paranoia, delusions, and hallucinations. He denies any side effects of the medications, has no abnormal movements, and is back to his baseline weight before taking olanzapine. When reviewing the medication's purpose, risks, and benefits, Mark initially stated, "I don't feel anything from it, so I don't see how it's working, but fine, I'll take it." He also said, "The fluoxetine helps me not get depressed, and this helps me not get manic; I guess I need them both." His mother prodded him, saying, "Remember, if you don't take this, you'll have to go back to the hospital." Mark agreed to be given the injection, and the FNP quickly gave it. She also gave him a refill for the fluoxetine. He and his mother then left the clinic and scheduled an appointment in four weeks when the next injection is due.

After Mark leaves, you ask the FNP whether it is acceptable to prescribe and administer medication like aripiprazole to a patient to treat bipolar disorder. Additionally, you believe that the patient reluctantly agreed to take the medication and wonder if the patient was somewhat coerced into being given the injection by his mother to avoid returning to the hospital. You also found it odd that a 26-year-old patient had their mother present with them at their visit. Lastly, you are concerned that no labs were ordered, as fasting blood glucose and a lipid profile should be checked one month after starting a second-generation antipsychotic such as aripiprazole (Scrandis, 2014).

Consider:

1. Identify the ethical concerns with this situation.

2. What information will you need before a responsible decision can be made? (Consider what the information is and where it will come from.)

3. Who are stakeholders involved in the decision, and what is the process in which those involved could come to a decision (e.g., what tools are/could be used to create an informed decision)?

4. What are the values relevant to this problem? *Values* are the things that you believe are important in making the decision. They (should) determine priorities. Values relevant to this problem may not be representative of your own personal values or moral framework.

5. What are the options for the decision? Think in terms of values and feasibility (e.g., financial, political, organizational, religious constraints).

Management of Case Study

After all considerations, write a short narrative of how you believe is the best way to manage this situation; list core values important to you for managing the situation.

References

Balestra, M. L. (2019). Family nurse practitioner scope of practice issues when treating patients with mental health issues. *The Journal for Nurse Practitioners*, *15*(7), 479–482. https://doi.org/10.1016/j.nurpra.2018.11.007

Scrandis, D. A. (2014). Identification and management of bipolar disorder. *The Nurse Practitioner*, *39*(10), 30–37. http://dx.doi.org/10.1097/01. NPR.0000453642.51780.97

DEPRESSION SCREENING IN ADOLESCENTS

Major depression is considered a serious mental health concern among adolescents, with far-reaching acute and chronic morbidity and mortality (Lu, 2019; Zuckerbrot et al., 2018). Untreated depression during adolescence can lead to negative social and health outcomes such as academic failure, violence, substance use, risky sexual behavior, suicidal behavior, and self-injurious behavior (Lu, 2019). Between 2011 and 2016, depression prevalence in adolescents increased from 8.3% to 12.9% (Lu, 2019). Additionally, the suicide rate for adolescents has risen, with a 56% increase between 2007 and 2018 (Centers for Disease Control and Prevention, 2020). In 2019, suicide was the second leading cause of death for individuals aged 10 to 24 (National Institute of Mental Health, n.d.). Despite increasing rates and significant negative outcomes associated with adolescent depression, 50% of adolescents with depression are not diagnosed prior to adulthood (Zuckerbrot et al., 2018). Moreover, even when diagnosed, only half of these adolescents receive appropriate treatment (Zuckerbrot et al., 2018).

Certain groups of adolescents are at an even higher risk of developing depression and the negative sequelae associated with it. Research has consistently demonstrated that transgender adolescents have increased rates of depression as well as suicidal thoughts and behaviors, self-injurious behaviors, and eating disorders when compared to cisgender adolescents (Connolly et al., 2016). Supported social transition and gender-affirming medical care have been demonstrated to improve psychological functioning and outcomes in transgender youth (Connolly et al., 2016).

Due to the shortage of specialty mental healthcare services for children and adolescents throughout the country, identification and management of depression by pediatricians in primary care are essential (Zuckerbrot et al., 2018). The American Academy of Pediatrics has developed updated clinical practice guidelines to guide providers in the identification, assessment, and initial management of depression, including screening and assessing for suicidal thoughts and safety planning if present (Zuckerbrot et al., 2018).

Depression Screening in Adolescents Case Study

You are a nurse practitioner student working with a family nurse practitioner (FNP) at a rural community health center. Today you are seeing a 14-year-old Caucasian male, Jake, for his well-child checkup, and he is brought in by his father. In reviewing his chart, you note that he plays football, has no concerning health history, but that at his appointment last year he screened positive for mild depression on the Patient Health Questionnaire 9 – Adolescent Version (PHQ–A) with a score of 8. At that time, he denied any suicidal thoughts. Anxiety was not screened for at his last visit. You could find no note of depression being discussed at his last checkup. Additionally, you note that Jake's mother has called the nurse a few times in the last two months saying that Jake is complaining of headaches and stomachaches frequently, which are causing him to miss school and football practice.

Today, you note that his PHQ-A score has increased to 14. Additionally, while he remains at the 75th percentile for height as he has throughout his life, his weight has dropped from the 70th percentile to the 50th percentile in the last year. Today, as Jake and his father walk in, his father is complaining about his long hair and asking him why he just doesn't cut it already. Jake appears uncomfortable in the room with his father, as if he is trying to get away from him. Jake is fidgety, making minimal eye contact and mostly looking at the floor. He initially answers questions monosyllabically or with grunts. The father reports that his only concerns regarding Jake's health are that he seems to be eating less and is trying to quit football, which he has played since he was 6. He also reports that Jake seems more withdrawn and irritable. When the FNP asks Jake why he no longer wants to play football, he shrugs, looks at the floor, and says he's just not interested in it anymore. His dad interjects and says he just needs to man up and try harder.

After Jake's father leaves the exam room, the FNP proceeds with the exam. The only abnormal findings are Jake's weight and his depression screening score. When the FNP discusses the PHQ-A score, Jake initially says he's fine, and then he begins crying and states he's so tired of "holding everything in and faking it all the time." After talking about what he means, he discloses that he thinks he's trans. He says he wants to quit football because he doesn't feel comfortable on the team anymore. He has told one of his close friends and his older sister who are accepting, but he is terrified to tell his parents, especially his dad. Jake says that both his parents are very religious and conservative and frequently make negative comments about LGBTQ people. He fears that if he comes out as trans to them, they will kick him out and he will be homeless. Jake acknowledges that he did complain to his mom about headaches and stomachaches because it would get him out of football and school. He hoped that if he had enough absences, he'd get kicked out of his Catholic school and have to go to public school.

The FNP discusses with Jake what he would like her to call him and which pronouns to use. He asks her to use male pronouns in his record and around his parents, so they do not find out. He also asks her not to tell his parents, especially his father, anything they discuss. The FNP agrees to not tell his parents about being trans; however, she does tell him that she will have to discuss his depression and treatment options with him and his father. Jake agrees with this approach. With Jake, she discusses counseling options, and Jake is amenable to this.

When his father returns to the room, the FNP lets him know that Jake's exam was normal except for his diminished weight and his depression. She recommends counseling for the depression and attributes his weight loss to his depression as well. The father asks if she can just give Jake a pill for the depression because they can't afford that counseling "nonsense" to talk about feelings. He also states that he'll work to push Jake to eat more. The FNP agrees to start Jake on Prozac 10mg daily. She counsels Jake and his father on side effects and instructs them to come back in three months to see how he is responding to the medication.

After Jake and his father leave, you ask the FNP why she didn't give Jake information on counseling services because as a 14-year-old in Oregon he is able to consent on his own for mental health treatment (Oregon Health Authority, 2016). She says that she wasn't going to recommend something that the parents weren't going to go along with. You also voice your concern that even though his depression was addressed, he wasn't screened for suicidal thoughts or an eating disorder. The FNP says she didn't ask about suicide because she doesn't know what to do if people say they are suicidal, because "the clinic doesn't have a policy about that."

Consider:

1. Identify the ethical concerns with this situation.

2. What information will you need before a responsible decision can be made? (Consider what the information is and where it will come from.)

3. Who are stakeholders involved in the decision, and what is the process in which those involved could come to a decision (e.g., what tools are/could be used to create an informed decision)?

4. What are the values relevant to this problem? *Values* are the things that you believe are important in making the decision. They (should) determine priorities. Values relevant to this problem may not be representative of your own personal values or moral framework.

5. What are the options for the decision? Think in terms of values and feasibility (e.g., financial, political, organizational, religious constraints).

Management of Case Study

After all considerations, write a short narrative of how you believe is the best way to manage this situation; list core values important to you for managing the situation.

References

Centers for Disease Control and Prevention. (2020, September 11). *State suicide rates among adolescents and young adults aged 10–24: United States, 2000–2018.* National Vital Statistics Reports, *69*(11) [PDF]. https://www.cdc.gov/nchs/data/nvsr/nvsr69/nvsr-69-11-508.pdf

Connolly, M. D., Zervos, M. J., Barone, C. J., Johnson, C. C., & Joseph, C. L. (2016). The mental health of transgender youth: Advances in understanding. *Journal of Adolescent Health, 59*(5), 489–495. https://doi.org/10.1016/j.jadohealth.2016.06.012

Lu, W. (2019). Adolescent depression: National trends, risk factors, and healthcare disparities. *American Journal of Health Behavior, 43*(1), 181–194. https://doi.org/10.5993/ajhb.43.1.15

National Institute of Mental Health. (n.d.). *Suicide.* Retrieved February 26, 2022, from https://www.nimh.nih.gov/health/statistics/suicide

Oregon Health Authority. (2016). *Minor rights: Access and consent to health care* [PDF]. https://www.oregon.gov/oha/PH/HEALTHYPEOPLEFAMILIES/ YOUTH/Documents/minor-rights.pdf

Zuckerbrot, R. A., Cheung, A., Jensen, P. S., Stein, R. E. K., Laraque, D., Levitt, A., Birmaher, B., Campo, J., Clarke, G., Emslie, G., Kaufman, M., Kelleher, K. J., Kutcher, S., Malus, M., Sacks, D., Waslick, B., & Sarvet, B. (2018). Guidelines for adolescent depression in primary care (GLAD-PC): Part I. Practice preparation, identification, assessment, and initial management. *Pediatrics, 141*(3), e20174081. https://doi.org/10.1542/peds.2017-4081

TREATMENT OF RESISTANT ANXIETY

Anxiety disorders are the most prevalent mental illness in the United States, impacting over 40 million adults aged 18 years and older every year (Anxiety & Depression Association of America [AADA], 2021). Anxiety disorders include agoraphobia, generalized anxiety disorder (GAD), panic disorder, selective mutism, separation anxiety disorder, social anxiety disorder, and specific phobia (American Psychiatric Association, 2013). Individuals with anxiety disorders experience a combination of psychological and somatic symptoms with varying presentations (Gregory & Hardy, 2022). Psychological symptoms of anxiety disorders include, but are not limited to, excessive worry, difficulty controlling worry, increased irritability, and difficulty concentrating, whereas the somatic symptoms may include tachycardia, feeling on edge, gastrointestinal distress, fatigue, insomnia, muscle tension, dry mouth, tremors, increased perspiration, and shortness of breath. Some individuals may experience a combination of psychological and somatic symptoms, whereas others may experience solely psychological or somatic symptoms (Gregory & Hardy, 2022). Anxiety disorders are highly treatable, yet only 37% of those suffering receive treatment

(AADA, 2021). Furthermore, many of those who do receive treatment receive inadequate treatment, with less than 20% of those receiving treatment that conforms with evidence-based guidelines (Roberge et al., 2015). GAD is the most prevalent anxiety disorder managed in the primary care setting (Ansara, 2020). Evidence-based treatment strategies for GAD may include first-line psychotherapy using cognitive behavioral therapy (CBT), cognitive therapy, or applied relaxation; first-line psychopharmacological intervention includes selective serotonin reuptake inhibitors (SSRIs) or serotonin norepinephrine reuptake inhibitors (SNRIs; AADA, 2016). *Treatment resistant anxiety* is often defined as lack of response to an antidepressant at an adequate dose for an adequate duration (Ansara, 2020; Patterson & Van Ameringen, 2016). It is recognized that response for anxiety disorders tends to take longer than that for depressive disorders; therefore, an adequate duration should be of eight weeks or longer at a therapeutic dose for anxiety, with known adherence, prior to considering treatment resistance.

Treatment of Resistant Anxiety Case Study

You are a psychiatric mental health nurse practitioner embedded in a patient-centered medical home. This is your second week on the job, and your position had been vacant for some time prior to you being hired. Additionally, there is a psychologist in the clinic as part of the team providing integrated behavioral healthcare to patients. It is your understanding that they are primarily available to provide short-term psychotherapy with interventions focused on health improvement, brief diagnostic evaluation for straightforward mental health issues, and assistance with referring out for more complex issues that require long-term management.

Today, you are seeing Carol, a 63-year-old woman with a past medical history significant for chronic obstructive pulmonary disease (COPD), obstructive sleep apnea (OSA), hypertension, hyperlipidemia, chronic low back pain, tobacco dependence in sustained remission, opiate dependence in sustained remission on buprenorphine/naloxone

maintenance therapy, insomnia, and treatment resistant anxiety. Her
current medications include nifedipine 60mg daily, simvastatin 20mg
daily, buprenorphine/naloxone 8mg/2mg BID, trazodone 100mg
nightly, clonazepam 2mg TID, and duloxetine 30mg daily. She has a
CPAP for her OSA but is documented to have poor adherence with
it as the mask "makes her anxious." This is your first time meeting
with Carol. Her family nurse practitioner (FNP) was able to touch
base with you briefly earlier in the day and explained that Carol was
prescribed the trazodone, duloxetine, and clonazepam by her previous
psychiatric provider and they are the "only regimen that works for her
treatment resistant anxiety." The FNP said he had significant safety
concerns regarding the combination of clonazepam, buprenorphine/
naloxone, and trazodone in a patient with COPD but that he had
agreed to "bridge" the patient with the medications until a new psychiatric provider was available as they were started by psychiatry, and
he felt the management of treatment resistant anxiety was outside of
his scope. As he was leaving the room, he made a comment about the
patient being extremely resistant to any discussion regarding medication changes or the risks inherent in her medications.

Carol is on time for her appointment with you, and she is pleasant
and polite. She appears quite fatigued overall and at one point does
doze off briefly. She reports that she slept poorly the night prior. She
describes her mood as "OK I guess, nervous." Her affect is reactive,
and she appears grossly euthymic. Her thoughts are linear and organized with no tangentiality or circumstantiality. She shows no evidence of delusional thought process, paranoia, or hallucinations and
denied suicidality. Carol reports she has been nervous for as "long as I
can remember, since I was a kid, I guess." She describes that she tends
to "worry about anything and everything," she feels uncomfortable
in crowds, often feels tense in her shoulders and neck, has difficulty
sleeping, and realizes her worried thoughts are often "unnecessary
or unrealistic" but can't stop them and will sometimes get so anxious
she can't eat. In high school and college, she drank alcohol to manage these feelings but stopped when a close friend died while driving
intoxicated. She rarely drinks alcohol now, but she feels much better
after a drink or two. After injuring her back at work in a factory about
15 years ago, she was prescribed oxycodone. She reports it helped

with the pain "a bit," but it really helped with the worry. Carol went on to describe how she became "addicted to the oxycodone and then heroin." She got sober when she lost her job due to her drug use and was able to get into treatment and has been on buprenorphine/naloxone for eight years after a heroin relapse. She denies that she has ever done any type of counseling other than attending Narcotics Anonymous meetings, which she reports are very helpful to her. She thinks she tried fluoxetine for her anxiety for two to three weeks 20 or so years ago but then she heard "about how it makes teenagers suicidal" and stopped taking it. After her back injury she was prescribed escitalopram 10mg daily, which she believes she took for approximately a year. She reports the escitalopram "didn't do a thing" for her anxiety, "but the oxycodone sure did; that's how I got hooked."

You review with Carol the risks associated with her current medication regimen, including increased respiratory depression and possible death due to the combination of buprenorphine/naloxone and clonazepam, which is further increased by trazodone along with her COPD and OSA. She listens carefully to everything you say and mentions that she recalls the pharmacist saying something about all that when she picked up her medications once and that it sounds serious. Carol says that her psychiatrist started her on the clonazepam when she was still using, and it helped her stick with treatment to get sober and none of those other medications ever worked. She goes on to say that after her psychiatrist retired and she started coming here for care, the last psychiatric provider continued these medications, and it didn't seem right for some new person who barely knows her to come in here and talk about changing them suddenly.

You review with Carol the evidence-based treatment guidelines for GAD, which include an SSRI or SNRI at an adequate dose for an adequate duration or psychotherapy such as CBT, either of which can be done alone or in combination with the other. You also explain that benzodiazepines, such as clonazepam, should only be used for short-term use, and that long-term use can worsen anxiety by causing rebound anxiety (Ansara, 2020). Additionally, her total daily dose of 6mg is above the recommended daily max of 4mg (AADA, 2016). Lastly, you explain that her current dose of duloxetine is not at a therapeutic dose to have efficacy for anxiety and recommend that it be increased to 60mg daily. You go on to recommend a slow, gradual taper of her clonazepam to decrease her risk of respiratory depression. You also recommend engagement with counseling and offer to take her to meet the psychologist in the clinic today to do a warm hand-over. Carol says she is willing to meet the psychologist to see what "all that is about" while expressing skepticism, as she already has a sponsor. She declines an increase in duloxetine as she knows that could increase her blood pressure and she doesn't "want to have a heart attack." In response to the suggestion to tapering the clonazepam, she appears angry and asks whether you had read her chart, saying, "The reason I take that much is because I have treatment resistant anxiety. Don't you know anything?"

Consider:

1. Identify the ethical concerns with this situation.

2. What information will you need before a responsible decision can be made? (Consider what the information is and where it will come from.)

3. Who are stakeholders involved in the decision, and what is the process in which those involved could come to a decision (e.g., what tools are/could be used to create an informed decision)?

4. What are the values relevant to this problem? *Values* are the things that you believe are important in making the decision. They (should) determine priorities. Values relevant to this problem may not be representative of your own personal values or moral framework.

5. What are the options for the decision? Think in terms of values and feasibility (e.g., financial, political, organizational, religious constraints).

Management of Case Study

After all considerations, write a short narrative of how you believe is the best way to manage this situation; list core values important to you for managing the situation.

References

American Psychiatric Association. (2013). *Diagnostic and statistical manual of mental disorders* (5th edition). American Psychiatric Publishing.

Ansara, E. D. (2020). Management of treatment-resistant generalized anxiety disorder. *Mental Health Clinician, 10*(6), 326–334. https://doi.org/10.9740/mhc.2020.11.326

Anxiety & Depression Association of America. (2016, March 16). *Clinical practice review for GAD.* https://adaa.org/resources-professionals/practice-guidelines-gad

Anxiety & Depression Association of America. (2021, September 19). *Understanding anxiety & depression.* Facts & statistics. https://adaa.org/understanding-anxiety/facts-statistics

Gregory, A., & Hardy, L. (2022, January 26). Anxiety in primary care: A primer for APRNs. *American Nurse Journal, 17*(2), 13–18. https://www.myamericannurse.com/anxiety-disorders-in-primary-care/

Patterson, B., & Van Ameringen, M. (2016). Augmentation strategies for treatment-resistant anxiety disorders: A systematic review and meta-analysis. *Depression and Anxiety, 33*(8), 728–736. https://doi.org/10.1002/da.22525

Roberge, P., Normand-Lauzière, F., Raymond, I., Luc, M., Tanguay-Bernard, M.-M., Duhoux, A., Bocti, C., & Fournier, L. (2015). Generalized anxiety disorder in primary care: Mental health services use and treatment adequacy. *BMC Family Practice, 16*(1). https://pubmed.ncbi.nlm.nih.gov/26492867/

COVID-19 VACCINE IN ADOLESCENCE

The benefit of childhood vaccination is well established. It has been said routine vaccination for communicable diseases was the single most significant achievement for the field of public health to come out of the 20th century (Rus & Groselj, 2021). However, over the last several decades, the ideas of "vaccine hesitancy," "vaccine reluctance," and "anti-vaccination" have become more prevalent than ever before, leading to lower numbers in childhood vaccination and allowing for diseases once thought eradicated to be reintroduced into society (Rus & Groselj, 2021). Fortunately, most current generations have not experienced how communicable diseases affected their ancestors before vaccination. Unfortunately, the shelter created by the high numbers of vaccinated people in past populations may, in part, be a cause of what has led to the decreased numbers in childhood vaccination today (Rus & Groselj, 2021).

In March 2020, the novel coronavirus (SARS-CoV-2 or COVID-19) made its way to America. As a result of the novel disease and its variants, just over a year later, in May 2021, it had infected over 150 million people and proved fatal for nearly 3.3 million people globally (World Health Organization, 2021). A vaccination against the disease was developed rapidly, and in May 2021, the vaccine received emergency use authorization from the US Food and Drug Administration to be given to adolescents aged 12 to 15 years (Center for Disease Control [CDC], 2020a). Despite significant data indicating the vaccine's safety and efficacy for this age group, parents and guardians remained hesitant or opposed to vaccinating their children.

Mercifully, most infected adolescents are spared from severe illness or death from COVID-19 (CDC, 2020a). Still, they pose serious concerns for public health officials, as this age group may not show symptoms, making it difficult to identify many COVID-19 cases in this population (CDC, 2020a). Regardless of being asymptomatic, adolescent children can still shed the virus and pass it along to the more vulnerable, such as the elderly or immunocompromised. Furthermore, children and adolescents who contract COVID-19 are at risk of developing multisystem inflammatory syndrome (MIS-C), a severe complication that may arise from the infection (CDC, 2020b). Children who develop MIS-C present with pervasive internal organ inflammation that may have a long-term effect on the heart, lungs, kidneys, brain, skin, etc. Current data show children who become fully vaccinated are less likely to become infected and spread the virus and do not typically become a target for MIS-C (CDC, 2020a, 2020b).

Ethics pertaining to adolescent vaccination are complex when a parent is not involved in the decision or disagrees with the adolescent on whether to get a vaccine. Principles from biomedical and public health ethics should be considered, along with the consideration of whether an adolescent has the capacity to make their own decisions (Silverman et al., 2019). Apart from a few US states, parental consent for vaccination is required for children and adolescents under the age of 18 (Kaiser Family Foundation, n.d.). Thus, most states require, by law, parental consent for vaccination, regardless of an adolescent's wishes. While the law is the authority by which medical professionals must practice, ethics and advocacy should also be considered when caring for a young person. Considering vaccination laws, the code of nursing ethics, and the ideals of autonomy, beneficence, and non-maleficence,

how can the advanced practice nurse be an advocate for their more
vulnerable adolescent patient?

COVID-19 Vaccine in Adolescence Case Study

You are a family nurse practitioner working for a family medicine
practice in Southern California. Today is a typical day in the office.
As you are going through your schedule with your assigned medical assistant (MA), you notice that you have an appointment with a
15-year-old boy, Barry, whom you have not seen before. The appointment note states that he "would like to discuss getting the COVID-19
vaccine." COVID-19 and the vaccines are something that everyone is
talking about at this time. New developments are happening daily, so
you are not surprised to see this type of appointment on your schedule. You are up to date and well versed in how the virus is transmitted
and statistics pertaining to severe illness and death. You also just read
an evidence-based, peer-reviewed article discussing the different
COVID-19 vaccines in question and how they have been proven safe
and effective for preventing major illness and death from COVID-19
for most of the population. Therefore, you look forward to providing
knowledge and insight into the vaccine for the patient and his parents.

When the patient arrives at the clinic, the MA brings him back, takes
his vital signs, and enters the chief complaint. Before you enter the
room, the MA flags you down quietly and whispers that the boy's parents are not with him, and he does not want them to know he is here.
You know that California law requires parental consent for vaccination and are concerned he may be expecting to get the vaccine today.
As you enter the room, you introduce yourself and ask Barry how he
is doing; he responds quickly, "Fine." In order to hear his concern in
his own words, you ask what brings him into the office today. He is
looking down at the floor when he responds in a low voice, "I wanna
talk about getting the COVID shot." You react to Barry by asking him
what exactly he would like to know and whether he has specific questions about the vaccine. He says to you, "I am scared I'm gonna get
COVID if I don't get the shot, but my dad won't let me get it because

he said that the government is putting microchips in it." He also relays to you that his best friend's father is ill with "some kind of cancer" and is not to be around people who are ill and are not vaccinated. After further discussion, you conclude that he has not been able to see his best friend in person in almost a year, and a driving force for wanting the vaccine is being able to reconnect with his friend in person. Barry continues by stating, "Nothing I tell my parents will make them listen to me." You explain to him the importance of becoming vaccinated and ease any fears he may have about the myth related to microchips in the vaccine. You begin to discuss vaccination laws for adolescents under 18 in California, and as you continue, Barry stops you and asks, "Can you just give me the shot today and not talk to my dad about it? He's just going to say no." He continues to explain that if you cannot provide the vaccine, he may as well leave because that is the only reason he is there. You realize that this is a more complex situation than you initially thought.

What do you do? How do you respond to Barry's question about whether you can give him the vaccine today?

Consider:

1. Identify the ethical concerns with this situation.

2. What information will you need before a responsible decision can be made? (Consider what the information is and where it will come from.)

3. Who are stakeholders involved in the decision, and what is the process in which those involved could come to a decision (e.g., what tools are/could be used to create an informed decision)?

4. What are the values relevant to this problem? *Values* are the things that you believe are important in making the decision. They (should) determine priorities. Values relevant to this problem may not be representative of your own personal values or moral framework.

5. What are the options for the decision? Think in terms of

values and feasibility (e.g., financial, political, organizational, religious constraints).

Management of Case Study

After all considerations, write a short narrative of how you believe is the best way to manage this situation; list core values important to you for managing the situation.

References

Centers for Disease Control and Prevention. (2020a, February 11). *Science brief: Transmission of SARS-CoV-2 in K-12 schools and early care and education programs – Updated*. https://www.cdc.gov/coronavirus/2019-ncov/science/science-briefs/transmission_k_12_schools.html

Centers for Disease Control and Prevention. (2020b, February 11). *Multisystem inflammatory syndrome in children (MIS-C) and adults (MIS-A)*. https://www.cdc.gov/mis/about.html

Kaiser Family Foundation. (n.d.). *State parental consent laws for COVID-19 vaccination*. https://www.kff.org/other/state-indicator/state-parental-consent-laws-for-covid-19-vaccination/?currentTimeframe=0&sortModel=%7B%22colId%22:%22Location%22,%22sort%22:%22asc%22%7D

Rus, M., & Groselj, U. (2021). Ethics of vaccination in childhood—A framework based on the four principles of biomedical ethics. *Vaccines, 9*(2), 113. https://doi.org/10.3390/vaccines9020113

Silverman, R. D., Opel, D. J., & Omer, S. B. (2019). Vaccination over parental objection—Should adolescents be allowed to consent to receiving vaccines? *New England Journal of Medicine, 381*(2), 104–106. https://doi.org/10.1056/nejmp1905814

World Health Organization. (2021, May 11). *Weekly epidemiological update on Covid-19 – 11 May 2021*. https://www.who.int/publications/m/item/weekly-epidemiological-update-on-covid-19---11-may-2021

10

CASE STUDY #11

MEDICAL EMANCIPATION VERSUS CONFIDENTIALITY IN TRANSGENDER AND GENDER-NONCONFORMING PEOPLE

Transgender and gender-nonconforming (TGNC) people are at a much greater risk of adverse physical and mental health outcomes when compared to their cisgender (a person who is not transgender) peers (Kimberly et al., 2018). TGNC individuals often suffer from anxiety and depression due to rejection from society, including family, friends, and even healthcare providers (Kimberly et al., 2018). They are also more likely to engage in activities that cause self-harm and are approximately 40 times more likely to attempt death by suicide (Dhejne et al., 2011; Grant et al., 2011).

Gender-affirming care from healthcare providers has demonstrated a largely positive effect on lessening the extent of these concerns (Kimberly et al., 2018). By providing support and affirmation for a person's gender identity, providers have the ability to adhere to the doctrines of beneficence and nonmaleficence. However, when managing these patients, a provider must consider several factors, such as access to knowledgeable care, affordability of gender-related treatments, and the permanent nature of certain treatment modalities, especially in children and adolescents who are TGNC (Kimberly et al., 2018). Thus, mindfulness for the principles of justice, beneficence, and nonmaleficence when treating these individuals should be considered.

Parents of adolescent TGNC individuals are not always open to the idea of their child's preferred gender identity if it is different from the one they were assigned at birth—especially those parents who come from a conservative background or are actively involved in a more conservative religion (Campbell et al., 2019). Campbell et al. (2019) discuss how active participation in certain religions is often linked with prejudice against TGNC people. They give the potential explanation: Religious people firmly believe they must adhere to rules, either written or spoken, against gender variation (Campbell et al., 2019). Thus, they tend to have a more negative attitude and nonacceptance toward the gender nonconforming (Campbell et al., 2019). Considering this information and the code of nursing ethics, the nurse practitioner must care for these individuals without judgment or bias and do what is in the best interest of the patient.

Medical Emancipation Versus Confidentiality Case Study

You are a family nurse practitioner working in rural Idaho for the last 10 years. You are one of two sole providers for the community. Today, it is a hot August day, and you will be seeing 27 patients with a variety of different medical and psychosocial concerns. It is not an atypical day for you to have several patients on your schedule belonging to the same family. As you are going over your schedule, you see the Clementine family is coming in for their school physicals and vaccinations.

Lisa, who is 18, graduated from high school in May and plans on attending Brigham Young University in the fall. Luna, 16 going on 17, attends the local high school, and Logan, 11, goes into middle school this coming fall. They are a lovely family and have a close relationship with each other and God. All the children are active in sports, and each Sunday, they attend the local ward at the Church of Jesus Christ of Latter-Day Saints. Looking back to their chart, it's been about two years since their last wellness exam; however, they have been seen for multiple acute concerns in that time. Also, the children's mother, Louisa, is a friend from church, so you have had the opportunity to see and get to know the children outside of the clinic setting. You know them as happy, outgoing, and active children, especially Luna; as long as you have known her, she is always playing some kind of sport. However, you noticed lately Luna has been more withdrawn at church than usual and are hoping to get some time to talk to her about how she is feeling at this potentially challenging point in her life. It comes time for the Clementines' appointments, and your medical assistant (MA) brings them back and gets their vital signs. After they are roomed, your MA approaches you and says, "I didn't even recognize Luna." She goes on and tells you Luna appears very tired, has lost weight, her BMI was 15.2, and she is noted to be in the 5th percentile on the growth chart. Her blood pressure was 94/56, pulse 106, and temperature 96.4. You see Lisa and Logan first, as you suspect you may spend a little extra time with Luna.

As you enter the room to see Luna, you notice she is withdrawn and is not looking you in the eye as you speak to her. On review of systems, she says she has no concerns; however, Louisa, her mom, states her periods have become erratic, and she has been complaining about headaches at least one to two days a week that keep her home from school. On physical exam, Luna appears slightly agitated, fidgety, pale, thin, and a bit disheveled. Louisa says Luna cut her hair short about a month ago because she decided she didn't want to deal with maintaining it anymore. She then states, "Teenagers are so lazy and weird." You continue with your physical exam and note that her heart rate is 102 and regular; you can easily visualize her skeletal structure when evaluating her for scoliosis and notice several small lacerations and scarring on the back of her upper arms. The rest of her physical exam is unremarkable.

As you do with all adolescents, you ask that Mom leave the room so you may have a conversation about more personal concerns. Mom says, "Of course," and leaves the room. You begin by letting Luna know whatever she tells you is confidential, and for you to give her the best possible care, she must be honest with you. You start with asking about current sexual activity, drugs, and alcohol, and she denies participation in these activities. You ask her how she is doing in school, and she becomes a bit tearful. She looks toward the ground and tells you she is not doing well because she has been missing school, and kids she has known since childhood have started to make fun of her because of her appearance. It's important that Luna feels comfortable and confident in talking to you about something so personal and often times embarrassing. In hope of displaying empathy for her, you share how you have worked with many young people who have been bullied and how you were personally bullied yourself as a child. She stops you and says, "Actually, it's not just about the bullying. I have always felt like something is wrong with me… like… I'm not a girl, I'm a guy, and I wanna be a guy. I wanna be able to cut my hair and play soccer with the boys; I want everyone to know me, not Luna." Luna goes on to tell you she has thought about talking with her mom but fears she will be rejected and will lose everyone and everything that means anything to her; additionally, she wouldn't be able to attend church, which is a large part of their family's life. "So please, you can't tell my mom, or I will die."

After more discussion, you come to find Luna had cut his hair because it makes him feel more "normal," and he has not been eating much because he read that if he loses enough weight, his periods might stop, and that should make him feel more like who he is. Luna then tells you he has been cutting himself on the back of his arms. It makes him feel better, as the pain feels better than how he normally feels. Unfortunately, you have no experience caring for transgender individuals and do not know anyone who does; plus, you don't feel this is right in the eyes of God. However, you know it is likely more harm will come to Luna if he does not get help. One of your largest concerns is Luna's weight loss and current BMI, likely because of not eating in hopes of amenorrhea. You discuss the possibility of starting a continuous birth control pill to stop the periods and ask if he would eat more if his periods were gone, and he says "yes." Unfortunately, you know Louisa would be completely against Luna starting birth control for any reason, so you struggle with whether this is the best thing to do.

With the information you have, how will you assist Luna in getting his needs met, and how will you keep him safe from further harm?

Consider:

1. Identify the ethical concerns with this situation.

2. What information will you need before a responsible decision can be made? (Consider what the information is and where it will come from.)

3. Who are stakeholders involved in the decision, and what is the process in which those involved could come to a decision (e.g., what tools are/could be used to create an informed decision)?

4. What are the values relevant to this problem? *Values* are the things that you believe are important in making the decision. They (should) determine priorities. Values relevant to this problem may not be representative of your own personal values or moral framework.

5. What are the options for the decision? Think in terms of values and feasibility (e.g., financial, political, organizational, religious constraints).

Management of Case Study

After all considerations, write a short narrative of how you believe is the best way to manage this situation; list core values important to you for managing the situation.

References

Campbell, M., Hinton, J. D. X., & Anderson, J. R. (2019). A systematic review of the relationship between religion and attitudes toward transgender and gender-variant people. *International Journal of Transgenderism, 20*(1), 21–38. https://doi.org/10.1080/15532739.2018.1545149

Dhejne, C., Lichtenstein, P., Boman, M., Johansson, A. L. V., Långström, N., & Landén, M. (2011). Long-term follow-up of transsexual persons undergoing sex reassignment surgery: Cohort study in Sweden. *PLoS ONE, 6*(2), e16885. https://doi.org/10.1371/journal.pone.0016885

Grant, J., Mottet, L., Tanis, J., Min, D., Harrison, J., Herma, J., & Keisling, M. (2011). *Injustice at every turn: A report of the national transgender discrimination survey.* https://transequality.org/sites/default/files/docs/resources/NTDS_Exec_Summary.pdf

Kimberly, L. L., Folkers, K. M., Friesen, P., Sultan, D., Quinn, G. P., Bateman-House, A., Parent, B., Konnoth, C., Janssen, A., Shah, L. D., Bluebond-Langner, R., & Salas-Humara, C. (2018). Ethical issues in gender-affirming care for youth. *Pediatrics, 142*(6). https://doi.org/10.1542/peds.2018-1537

CHILDHOOD OBESITY

The global burden of obesity continues to worsen. The World Health Organization (WHO) estimated that in 2017, more than 4 million people died from being overweight or obese (WHO, 2022). The number of overweight or obese people worldwide continues to grow, with the prevalence in children 5–19 years old increasing from 4% to 18% (WHO, 2022). Historically, being overweight or obese was a condition found in developed countries but now is also seen more in low- and middle-income countries (WHO, 2022).

In the United States, one in five children is obese. Childhood obesity increases the risk for serious health consequences, including respiratory problems, fractures, hypertension, and insulin resistance (Centers for Disease Control and Prevention [CDC], 2022). Children who are obese have a higher risk of suffering from depression, reduced quality of life scores, poor self-esteem, and emotional and behavioral problems (Rankin et al., 2016). Overweight and obese children frequently experience stigma, teasing, and bullying about their weight (Rankin et al., 2016). Finally, being overweight or obese in childhood increases the chance of obesity and premature death in adulthood (CDC, 2022). Childhood obesity impacts populations disproportionately, with Hispanic children having a higher prevalence of 25.6%, non-Hispanic Black children 24.2%, non-Hispanic White children 16.1%, and non-Hispanic Asian children 8.7% (CDC, 2022).

The causes of obesity are multifactorial. Solutions must therefore be both individualized and comprehensive. The most common cause of being overweight or obese is an energy imbalance of too many calories consumed and too few calories expended through activity (WHO, 2022). The environment in which people live also plays a crucial role in supporting people's likelihood of maintaining a healthy weight (CDC, 2022). Consider not having safe outdoor spaces or sidewalks to support easy access to physical activity. Food portions have increased significantly, making even more physical activity necessary to maintain a healthy weight. Many people live in food deserts and don't have easy access to affordable healthy foods, such as fresh fruits and vegetables. Food advertising encourages people to buy unhealthy foods and sugary drinks (CDC, 2022). Genetics, health conditions, medications, stress, and poor sleeping routines can also contribute to an increased risk of being overweight or obese (CDC, 2022).

Healthcare organizations and public health policy leaders have implemented nationwide programs, providing recommendations and resources designed to decrease the number of overweight and obese children. While there has been a recent plateau in the numbers of overweight and obese children, more needs to be done to improve universal health and mitigate the risks of childhood obesity (University of Washington, Department of Bioethics and Humanities, 2018).

One point of view is that parents should be held responsible for their child's weight and health, especially because obesity is known to be a condition of harm (Holms, 2010). Research suggests that while talking about unhealthy weight gain, nutrition, and physical activity with parents can help mitigate the risk of childhood obesity, many providers are reluctant to initiate these discussions. Reasons for not having this conversation include busy clinic schedules, lack of interdisciplinary support, providers' concern about a parent's reaction, or the parent's denial of a child's increasing weight and health consequences (Feiring et al., 2020). Also, providers may not have confidence in their communication and coaching skills in supporting parents to make positive nutritional and activity changes with and for their children (Regber et al., 2013).

Obese Child Case Study

You are a family nurse practitioner working in a busy urban health clinic serving a low-income, underinsured population in Los Angeles, California. You have a busy schedule today and are seeing 10-year-old Isaac, who is here with his mother, Gloria. Isaac is here for a routine well-child exam/sports physical. You have not seen Isaac in two years, when you first noted that he was overweight and his weight was trending upward. At that time, you discussed nutrition and activity with Gloria, who did not see her son's weight as a problem. She was angry that you brought it up as a concern. Your clinic has comprehensive services, so you referred him to the nutritionist but see that he and his mother never kept the appointment. In the review of his chart today, you note that Isaac is 56 inches in height and weighs 102 pounds. You calculate his BMI and find that it is in the 96th percentile.

You enter the exam room and greet Isaac and his mother. Gloria states Isaac has not had any illnesses, ER visits, or hospitalizations since you last saw him and that he is feeling well although mentions he can't keep up with his classmates during recess. You update his history, asking questions about his academic performance, his participation in activities at school and home, and how the family is doing as well. You perform a physical examination to find everything within normal limits for his age and development except his weight. You begin to discuss Isaac's weight, and Gloria breaks down and starts to cry. She states she has tried to have her son eat more fruits and vegetables and be more active. "He won't listen to me, and he eats what he wants. I worry that he will get fatter and get diabetes like his father." Isaac seems unconcerned and just wants you to sign his form so he can play baseball this spring. Meanwhile the medical assistant taps on your door to let you know that you are behind on your schedule and that your next patient is waiting.

With your knowledge of childhood obesity and its consequences, how would/could you respond to Gloria?

Consider:

1. Identify the ethical concerns with this situation.

2. What information will you need before a responsible decision can be made? (Consider what the information is and where it will come from.)

3. Who are stakeholders involved in the decision, and what is the process in which those involved could come to a decision (e.g., what tools are/could be used to create an informed decision)?

4. What are the values relevant to this problem? *Values* are the things that you believe are important in making the decision. They (should) determine priorities. Values relevant to this problem may not be representative of your own personal values or moral framework.

5. What are the options for the decision? Think in terms of values and feasibility (e.g., financial, political, organizational, religious constraints).

Management of Case Study

After all considerations, write a short narrative of how you believe is the best way to manage this situation; list core values important to you for managing the situation.

References

Centers for Disease Control and Prevention. (2022). *Overweight & obesity*. https://www.cdc.gov/obesity/

Feiring, E., Traina, G., Fystro, J. R., & Hofmann, B. (2020). Avoiding hypersensitive reluctance to address parental responsibility in childhood obesity. *Journal of Medical Ethics*, *48*, 65–69. https://jme.bmj.com/content/48/1/65

Holms, S. (2010). Cause and consequence. Parental responsibility and childhood obesity. In V. S. Vandamme, S. van de Vathorst, & I. de Beaufort, *Whose weight is it anyway? Essays on ethics & eating* (pp. 93–104). https://books.google.com/ books?id=IxRejWFie6wC&pg=PA93&source=gbs_toc_r&cad=4#v=onepage&q&f=false

Rankin, J., Matthews, L., Cobley, S., Han, A., Sanders, R., Wiltshire, H. D., & Baker, J. S. (2016). Psychological consequences of childhood obesity: Psychiatric comorbidity and prevention. *Adolescent Health, Medicine and Therapeutics*, *7*, 125–146.

Regber, S., Mårild, S., & Johansson Hanse, J. (2013). Barriers to and facilitators of nurse-parent interaction intended to promote healthy weight gain and prevent childhood obesity at Swedish child health centers. *BMC Nursing*, *12*(1), 1–11. https://doi.org/10.1186/1472-6955-12-27

University of Washington, Department of Bioethics and Humanities. (2018). *Public health ethics: Case 4*. https://depts.washington.edu/bhdept/ethics-medicine/bioethics-topics/cases/public-health-ethics-case-4

World Health Organization. (2022). *Obesity*. https://www.who.int/health-topics/obesity#tab=tab_1

12

DEMENTIA AND STOPPING DRIVING

As the population ages, rates of cognitive impairment will also increase. While aging is often associated with cognitive decline, not all older adults experience cognitive impairment. It is estimated that 10–15% of older adults in primary care show evidence of cognitive impairment, though estimates in studies vary due to differing definitions (Holsinger et al., 2012). Cognitive impairment is often overlooked in busy primary care practices, and once identified, providers often struggle to make recommendations that ethically balance safety and independence, such as whether to curtail driving (Aronson, 2019; Holsinger et al., 2012).

Primary care providers (PCPs) are responsible for assisting their patients with maximizing their health and functioning, thus assisting patients in maintaining their independence. Driving is essential in helping older adults maintain their independence. Losing the ability to drive results in dependence upon others and is also a concrete representation of many of the losses people experience as they age. Making the decision to stop driving is difficult and often occurs in the context of an acute medical condition or after a motor vehicle crash and can be made by an individual, their family, or a medical provider (Pozzi et al., 2017). PCPs may hesitate to take the steps necessary to remove a patient's driving privileges because they do not feel they have the expertise necessary to make the recommendation, they don't want to make the patient angry, or they worry that removing their driving privileges may harm their health and well-being. Determining how to move forward in these situations can be challenging when the risks are not necessarily clear.

Dementia and Stopping Driving Case Study

You are a family nurse practitioner in a busy primary care office. Janet, an 81-year-old widow with past medical history significant for hypertension (HTN), hyperlipidemia (HLD), diabetes mellitus type 2 (DM2), obstructive sleep apnea (OSA), bilateral cataract surgery approximately six years ago, anxiety, and mild cognitive impairment (MCI), is seen for followup with her son as she has just returned to her home after being admitted to the hospital and then a skilled nursing facility (SNF). Nearly two months ago, she tripped while golfing and fractured her right hip, which required surgery. Her hospital course was complicated by post-surgical delirium. Delirium initially improved with reduction in opioids; however, she then developed a urinary tract infection (UTI), causing a reemergence of delirium. After treatment with antibiotics and discontinuation of opioids, her mental status improved. She participated in physical therapy and was discharged to the SNF for ongoing rehab. Her son is concerned because he recalls a doctor in the hospital telling him that "it probably isn't safe for Janet to drive anymore" and referenced some cognitive testing that she scored poorly on. He didn't recall her score or which cognitive test it was. He did recall that they scanned her head because her behavior was so "wild," but everything was "fine." As he is telling you all this, Janet is becoming visibly frustrated. She interrupts and says, "My behavior wasn't that bad! I was confused because of all those pain meds and that darn infection!" She then insists, "I think I can drive just fine. I'm getting along all right now on my own. I'm just a little slower on my feet, that's all!" She then turns to her son and says, "What, are you going to drive me around everywhere I need to go? You're busy working all the time. I've been stuck at home all alone since you wouldn't let me drive until we came and talked about this here." It becomes clear to you that Janet is concerned about the isolation and loss of independence she is experiencing and that her son is concerned about her safety.

In reviewing Janet's records, you see that she completed a Montreal Cognitive Assessment (MoCA) three months prior to breaking her hip and scored a 24, indicating MCI (Nasreddine, 2022). This represents a one-point reduction from her previous score two years prior. Her HTN, HLD, DM2, and anxiety have been well controlled for years with chlorthalidone, amlodipine, atorvastatin, metformin, and citalopram. She uses a CPAP machine for her OSA and has good adherence, as demonstrated by data uploaded from the machine to her electronic medical record (EMR). When last seen, she declined starting a cholinesterase inhibitor for MCI because she did not find her cognitive issues troubling enough to add additional medications. She has been noted to have issues whenever given narcotic pain medications in the past, including confusion and hallucinations. Janet has not missed any routine appointments with you for the last few years. She uses the messaging function in the EMR appropriately and has gone to specialists when referred. She was approximately 15 minutes late for an appointment nine months ago because she got lost on the way to the clinic. The clinic had moved to a new building about three miles from where it had been previously, and Janet had only been to the new building one time. Since cataract surgery, she has only needed readers. No recent vision or hearing testing is available. Janet can hear you when you speak in a slightly louder than conversational tone. You did overhear her son complaining about how loud she turned the radio up in the car while he was driving her to the appointment.

From her hospital admission records, you can see that a MoCA was completed during her admission; she scored 15, indicating moderate cognitive impairment. Additionally, her head computed tomography (CT) scan that her son referenced showed no acute intracranial findings, along with mild generalized atrophy consistent with her age. The

MoCA was completed on the day she started antibiotics for her UTI, and no repeat cognitive testing was done in the hospital or SNF. Some medication changes were made during her hospitalization due to her acute condition, but by the time of discharge from the SNF, she had returned to her previous dosages of the medications she was maintained on previously to manage her chronic conditions.

Janet values her independence, her friendships with the women from church, her volunteer groups, and her golf, garden, and bridge clubs. Since the death of her husband eight years ago, she has maintained an active lifestyle with no plans on slowing down. Janet has made some modifications with the help of her children over the last eight years. Her children are designated medical and financial powers of attorney in the event she becomes incapacitated. Her daughter helped her set up online bill pay so her bills are paid automatically. She orders her groceries online and has them delivered to her home or her car in the store parking lot to avoid navigating the store with her cart and having to carry the bags. This habit proved quite helpful during the COVID-19 pandemic. When golfing, she uses a driving cart rather than a walking cart for her clubs and has someone at the course get her clubs out of her trunk for her. She stores her clubs in the trunk of her car to avoid having to lift them at home. Finally, her medications are delivered from the pharmacy in bubble packs, so she doesn't have to pack a weekly pill box. Despite this, she is still able to list the names, dosages, and purposes of her medications.

Since discharge from the SNF a week ago, Janet's son has been keeping her car keys to prevent her from driving based upon the recommendation of the hospital. This has been a significant source of conflict and frustration between them. Janet is hoping to sort it out with you today and resume driving. She insists that she hasn't had a ticket since she was a teenager and has not been in any crashes, so she must be safe to drive. You know that there are many benefits to extending a senior's ability to drive such as improved social connectedness, independence, prevention of isolation, and facilitation of access to nutrition, healthcare, and other services (American Geriatrics Society [AGS], 2020).

To assess safety in an older driver, you know you need to consider a patient's vision, cognitive, and functional status at a minimum (AGS, 2020). Risk factors for unsafe driving in older adults include polypharmacy (> 5 drugs), driving < 60 miles per week, deficits in cognitive functioning or attention, presence of a sleep disorder, hearing impairment or vision disturbance, alcohol abuse, caregiver concern about driving, lacking function in two or more activities of daily living, and a history of two or more traffic citations in the past three years (Pozzi et al., 2017). You don't think it is possible to complete a thorough assessment to evaluate Janet for risk factors for unsafe driving as well as complete the other necessary tasks of your follow-up visit with Janet. Based upon her ability to engage in the visit and describe her recent medical and life events, it appears that Janet's cognition has improved from what you would expect based on the MoCA testing completed in the hospital—though you have no evidence to support that and may be wrong. She is ambulating independently with a cane; she appears weak and readily acknowledges that she is slower than typical. You haven't assessed her strength and flexibility in her right leg as she is post-fracture, surgery, and rehab. It is clear you do not have enough information to make a definitive decision regarding her driver safety. Furthermore, you practice in a state with mandated reporting of unsafe drivers to the department of motor vehicles (DMV; Aronson, 2019). Janet's son does not know if a report was made to the DMV.

Consider:

1. Identify the ethical concerns with this situation.

2. What information will you need before a responsible decision can be made? (Consider what the information is and where it will come from.)

3. Who are stakeholders involved in the decision, and what is the process in which those involved could come to a decision (e.g., what tools are/could be used to create an informed decision)?

4. What are the values relevant to this problem? *Values* are the things that you believe are important in making the decision. They (should) determine priorities. Values relevant to this problem may not be representative of your own personal values or moral framework.

5. What are the options for the decision? Think in terms of values and feasibility (e.g., financial, political, organizational, religious constraints).

Management of Case Study

After all considerations, write a short narrative of how you believe is the best way to manage this situation; list core values important to you for managing the situation.

References

American Geriatrics Society. (2020). *Clinician's guide to assessing and counseling older drivers* (4th ed.). https://geriatricscareonline.org/application/content/products/B047/pdf/Clinicians_Guide_to_Assessing_and_Counseling_Older_Drivers_Feb_2020.pdf

Aronson, L. (2019). Don't ruin my life — Aging and driving in the 21st century. *New England Journal of Medicine, 380*(8), 705–707. https://doi.org/10.1056/nejmp1613342

Holsinger, T., Plassman, B. L., Stechuchak, K. M., Burke, J. R., Coffman, C. J., & Williams, J. W. (2012). Screening for cognitive impairment: Comparing the performance of four instruments in primary care. *Journal of the American Geriatrics Society, 60*(6), 1027–1036. https://doi.org/10.1111/j.1532-5415.2012.03967.x

Nasreddine, Z. (2022). *FAQ: MoCA – Cognitive Assessment.* https://www.mocatest.org/faq/

Pozzi, C., Lucchi, E., Lanzoni, A., Gentile, S., Morghen, S., Trabucchi, M., Bellelli, G., & Morandi, A. (2017). Why older people stop to drive? A cohort study of older patients admitted to a rehabilitation setting. *Aging Clinical and Experimental Research, 30*(5), 543–546. https://doi.org/10.1007/s40520-017-0804-x

WHEN TO TRANSITION TO PALLIATIVE CARE

Living with serious illness is a complex journey that requires patients and their loved ones to navigate potentially distressing symptoms, fragmented healthcare, and significant uncertainty. Palliative care has emerged in the last 30 years as a specialized interdisciplinary approach to help improve quality of life for populations facing serious illness (Center to Advance Palliative Care [CAPC], 2020; Institute of Medicine, 2014). As medical and technological innovations have prolonged survival for diagnoses that were previously considered significantly life-limiting, palliative care can support the physical, psychosocial, and spiritual needs of patients and caregivers. Engaging palliative care providers in patient care across the trajectory of serious illness has led to improvements in quality measures and resource utilization throughout the healthcare system (CAPC, 2020; Singer et al., 2016).

Communication is a critical skill in palliative care because eliciting patient goals and values helps support decision-making. Clinicians have historically advocated for advance care planning to help patients identify wishes for the care they wish to receive at the end of life (Zhou et al., 2010). In the context of serious illness, assessing a patient's understanding of their current health condition is an important initial step so that they can make informed choices about their care. Advance care planning also involves recording these preferences so that they can be honored by healthcare providers, ideally in any setting (Hospice & Palliative Nurses Association, 2011). Documentation via advance directives or living wills provides clarification about where and how patients wish to receive care at the end of life and identifies a healthcare proxy to speak on their behalf.

As palliative care continues to be integrated throughout the healthcare system, measures for success have been developed (Dy et al., 2015; Weissman et al., 2010). The National Consensus Project for Quality Palliative Care (NCP) was established in 2001 to identify standards for palliative care clinical programs (Meier, 2010), and evidence-based guidelines were updated in 2018 (NCP, 2018). Quality indicators related to palliative care include measures of advance directive completion (National Committee for Quality Assurance, 2020; NCP, 2018). Healthcare providers can also bill for the time spent discussing goals of care and advance care planning with patients (Medicare Learning Network, 2020).

Palliative care clinicians and researchers have recently questioned the conventional wisdom behind advance care planning, arguing that documenting these discussions as a "one and done" clinical benchmark oversimplifies the nuanced and iterative nature of conversations about end-of-life preferences (Jacobsen et al., 2022). Identifying patients' wishes should not rely on a single document but instead should involve ongoing conversations in the specific context of a patient and their illness trajectory.

When to Transition to Palliative Care Case Study

You are a nurse practitioner working in a busy cancer center affiliated with a research institute. Many of the oncologists are involved with phase one clinical trials for patients who have progressed through multiple lines of treatment. Your role in the clinic is to provide consultation as a palliative care specialist. One of the patients you recently met is a 22-year old woman, Katie, with colorectal cancer that has metastasized to her liver. She has undergone multiple lines of chemotherapy and has recently transferred care to your clinic to enroll in a clinical trial. When you meet her initially, she has multiple physical symptoms that are causing her considerable distress, so the focus of your first few visits is on alleviating her discomfort. She mentions feeling anxious about her worsening disease but states that usually when she worries about her mortality or her well-being, she "talks to herself" and is able to feel better. Katie is estranged from her parents and lives with her cousin and his partner. She works full-time at an acupuncture clinic and feels well-supported by her employer, but she is worried that the clinical trial will force her to take medical leave if she does not tolerate the side effects. You start to explore advance directives with her, but she has not identified a healthcare proxy and wants more time to think about it. You plan to follow up in two weeks once the clinical trial has started.

One week later, you hear from your team's social worker that Katie was found unresponsive at home and taken to the hospital. A brain MRI revealed a large brain metastasis surrounded by significant edema, causing a midline shift and likely to herniate in the next few days. Her cousin is the only family member the medical team can locate, and he makes the difficult decision to focus on comfort care, but the next day she starts to respond to painful stimuli. According to the intensivists, it is believed that strong intravenous steroids decreased the edema in her brain and allowed her condition to improve somewhat, but there is disagreement on the medical team about how to proceed. A neurosurgeon offers to attempt resection of the brain met, knowing that without intervention, her brain will still herniate, leading to her certain death. The oncologist overseeing her clinical trial points out that Katie's disease has progressed through multiple lines of treatment, and she would be ineligible to continue the trial because of her brain met, so she would have no other systemic treatment options. A different oncologist points out that because she is otherwise young and healthy and has no end-organ damage, resection of the tumor could prolong her survival and give her time to be eligible for future clinical trials.

In the meantime, Katie's cousin has been able to contact her estranged parents, and they arrive at the hospital distraught about their daughter's condition. Because Katie had not yet completed an advance directive, there is uncertainty among family members about what her wishes would be. Her parents disagree with each other about how to proceed. One parent wants to continue comfort care, pointing out that because her cancer is so aggressive, it would only get worse while she was recovering from surgery and likely result in a prolonged and more painful death than if she died of a brain herniation. The other parent argues that "she has always been a fighter" and points out that she is too young to let her die without trying to save her first. They argue that if she has more time, there may be another treatment option for her in the future.

As the palliative care provider who has worked with Katie most recently, you are invited by the intensive care team to a family meeting to share what you have learned about her and try to help the family come to a decision.

Consider:

1. Identify the ethical concerns with this situation.

2. What information will you need before a responsible decision can be made? (Consider what the information is and where it will come from.)

3. Who are stakeholders involved in the decision, and what is the process in which those involved could come to a decision (e.g., what tools are/could be used to create an informed decision)?

4. What are the values relevant to this problem? *Values* are the things that you believe are important in making the decision. They (should) determine priorities. Values relevant to this problem may not be representative of your own personal values or moral framework.

5. What are the options for the decision? Think in terms of values and feasibility (e.g., financial, political, organizational, religious constraints).

Management of Case Study

After all considerations, write a short narrative of how you believe is the best way to manage this situation; list core values important to you for managing the situation.

References

Center to Advance Palliative Care. (2020). *About palliative care.* https://www.capc.org/about/palliative-care/

Dy, S. M., Kiley, K. B., Ast, K., Lupu, D., Norton, S. A., McMillan, S. C., Herr, K., Rotella, J. D., & Casarett, D. J. (2015). Measuring what matters: Top-ranked quality indicators for hospice and palliative care from the American Academy of Hospice and Palliative Medicine and Hospice and Palliative Nurses Association. *Journal of Pain and Symptom Management, 49*(4), 773–781. https://doi.org/10.1016/j.jpainsymman.2015.01.012

Hospice & Palliative Nurses Association. (2011). HPNA position statement: The nurse's role in advance care planning. *Journal of Hospice & Palliative Nursing, 13*(4), 199–201. https://doi.org/10.1097/NJH.0b013e3182230a2b

Institute of Medicine. (2014). *Dying in America: Improving quality and honoring individual preferences near the end of life.* The National Academies Press.

Jacobsen, J., Bernacki, R., & Paladino, J. (2022). Shifting to serious illness communication. *JAMA, 327*(4), 321–322. https://doi.org/10.1001/jama.2021.23695

Medicare Learning Network. (2020). *Advance care planning* [Fact sheet]. https://www.cms.gov/outreach-and-education/medicare-learning-network-mln/mlnproducts/downloads/advancecareplanning.pdf

Meier, D. E. (2010). The development, status, and future of palliative care. In D. E. Meier, S. L. Isaacs, & R. G. Hughes (Eds.), *Palliative care: Transforming the care of serious illness* (pp. 3–76). Jossey-Bass. http://www.rwjf.org/content/dam/farm/books/books/2010/rwjf57523

National Committee for Quality Assurance. (2020). *Quality measure: Advance care plan.* National Quality Forum. https://www.qualityforum.org/QPS/MeasureDetails.aspx?standardID=291&print=1&entityTypeID=1

National Consensus Project for Quality Palliative Care. (2018). *Clinical practice guidelines for quality palliative care* (4th ed.). National Coalition for Hospice & Palliative Care. https://www.nationalcoalitionhpc.org/ncp

Singer, A. E., Goebel, J. R., Kim, Y. S., Dy, S. M., Ahluwalia, S. C., Clifford, M., Dzeng, E., O'Hanlon, C. E., Motala, A., Walling, A. M., Goldberg, J., Meeker, D., Ochotorena, C., Shanman, R., Cui, M., & Lorenz, K. A. (2016). Populations and interventions for palliative and end-of-life care: A systematic review. *Journal of Palliative Medicine, 19*(9), 995–1008. https://doi.org/10.1089/jpm.2015.0367

Weissman, D. E., Morrison, R. S., & Meier, D. E. (2010). Center to Advance Palliative Care palliative care clinical care and customer satisfaction metrics consensus recommendations. *Journal of Palliative Medicine, 13*(2), 179–184. https://doi.org/10.1089/jpm.2009.0270

Zhou, G., Stoltzfus, J. C., Houldin, A. D., Parks, S. M., & Swan, B. A. (2010). Knowledge, attitudes, and practice behaviors of oncology advanced practice nurses regarding advanced care planning for patients with cancer. *Oncology Nursing Forum, 37*(6), E400–410.

PRESCRIPTION REFILL DILEMMA FOR PATIENT AND SPOUSE IN FINANCIAL STRAITS

Prescription drug prices in the United States have created substantial challenges for patients and healthcare providers (Tsou et al., 2021). Drug prices can have an impact on how a patient is cared for, such as limiting access to certain treatments; this may impact the quantity and velocity in which disease states affect a patient or population (Tsou et al., 2021). In other words, prescription drug prices pose serious challenges to the fair distribution of benefits and burdens of disease in the general public (Tsou et al., 2021).

More specifically, medications that assist in lowering a diabetic patient's glucose have become one of the most expensive medication groups in America, and the prices continue to rise. According to Taylor (2020), healthcare expenditures for these medications increased by 240% from $16.9 billion in 2005–2007 to $57.6 billion per year in 2015–2017. Unfortunately, this financial burden has a devastating impact on people who do not have health insurance or for those with plans that come with high deductibles (Taylor, 2020). Thus, the high cost of these medications has significant implications for public policy and social justice (Taylor, 2020).

The American Nurses Association Code of Ethics provides guidelines for working through healthcare expense challenges in a legal, safe, and ethical way. Provisions of the code allow nurses to use their own judgment and critical thinking skills to provide fair and equitable care for their patients, whether it be an individual, family, group, community, or population, while still upholding the principles of nursing ethics (Haddad & Geiger, 2018). The Code of Ethics directs nurses to ensure they minimize harm and promote good for their patients as well as provide unprejudiced care regardless of a patient's socioeconomic status, race, sexual orientation, or age (Haddad & Geiger, 2018).

Refill Case Study

You are a nurse practitioner working in a family medicine/urgent care clinic in North Carolina. Today you are seeing Tony, a Caucasian man who just turned 65 years old. He has been your patient since you began practicing five years ago. You also see his wife, Marline, although it has been almost a year since you have seen either of them until today. They both have complicated medical histories, so you have been trying to get them in for a follow-up appointment for quite some time.

It is likely Tony is presenting today because you declined to fill any of his medications until he came in for a follow-up appointment and blood work. Tony has a long past medical history, including coronary artery disease, hypertension, diabetes with polyneuropathy, degenerative disc disease, anxiety, and depression, among others. He presents to the clinic for his welcome to Medicare annual wellness exam. As you enter the room and greet him, he shares he has just retired from 40 years as a construction worker for a large development firm. He tells you he "just couldn't do it anymore." You congratulate him on his retirement, and he tells you he wanted to "hang on for one more year" so that Marline would have insurance coverage until she was

65. Still, the stress and physical impact of the job had begun to take a severe toll on his mental and physical health. With the degenerative disc disease and polyneuropathy, Tony has been struggling with pain and the ability to walk for any length of time for several years now. Unfortunately, he shares that he is not in the best financial situation and tells you he is very stressed over how he and Marline are going to get by with her not working and just his Social Security money for income. You complete his physical exam and notify him of what he is due to have done.

Tony takes several prescriptions that he needs to be refilled today. The medications include metformin 1000mg twice daily and insuline glargine 60 units daily for his diabetes, duloxetine for his polyneu-ropathy and anxiety and depression, and lisinopril and metoprolol for his coronary artery disease and hypertension. You are getting ready to write his prescriptions when he stops you and says, "Is there any way you could double the prescriptions for metformin and insuline glargine? You know, Marline takes these medications too. Also, could you write a prescription for me for the other diabetes medication Marline takes? I think it's called Januvia. I am so embarrassed. But we just can't afford them for both of us right now. It won't be forever I promise. If you can't, I will have to share my prescriptions with her, which is fine, but I won't be able to take them as you want me to, and she will have to stop that other prescription she takes too." You know it is wrong and illegal to write prescriptions for a person under some-one else's name. However, you are torn and think to yourself how much you want to help them in their situation. You also know that Marline cannot physically afford to be without her diabetic medica-tions, as her last HbA1c was 8.7. She was also diagnosed several years ago by her therapist with a severe panic disorder that at one point had led to a hospital admission. The diazepam helps with calming her in acute episodes of panic.

Considering these people are both your patients and under your care, how will you proceed with Tony's request?

Consider:

    1. Identify the ethical concerns with this situation.

2. What information will you need before a responsible decision can be made? (Consider what the information is and where it will come from.)

3. Who are stakeholders involved in the decision, and what is the process in which those involved could come to a decision (e.g., what tools are/could be used to create an informed decision)?

4. What are the values relevant to this problem? *Values* are the things that you believe are important in making the decision. They (should) determine priorities. Values relevant to this problem may not be representative of your own personal values or moral framework.

5. What are the options for the decision? Think in terms of values and feasibility (e.g., financial, political, organizational, religious constraints).

Management of Case Study

After all considerations, write a short narrative of how you believe is the best way to manage this situation; list core values important to you for managing the situation.

References

Haddad, L. M., & Geiger, R. A. (2018). *Nursing ethical considerations*. StatPearls Publishing. http://europepmc.org/books/NBK526054

Taylor, S. I. (2020). The high cost of diabetes drugs: Disparate impact on the most vulnerable patients. *Diabetes Care, 43*(10), 2330–2332. https://doi.org/10.2337/dci20-0039

Tsou, A. Y., Graf, W. D., Russell, J. A., & Epstein, L. G. (2021). Ethical perspectives on costly drugs and health care. *Neurology, 97*(14), 685–692. https://doi.org/10.1212/wnl.0000000000012571

CRNA LABOR AND DELIVERY EPIDURAL PAIN MANAGEMENT WITH A LANGUAGE BARRIER

You are a certified registered nurse anesthetist (CRNA) at a large metropolitan teaching hospital assigned to a weekend 24-hour shift in the childbirth unit. Your duties are to provide coverage for labor-delivery neuraxial analgesia, caesarean section (C-section), urgent emergent care, and intravenous (IV) starts. The CRNA must be available for backup coverage for anesthesiology residents covering the main operating room and be available for codes, emergency intubations, blood patches, cardioversions, and placement of arterial lines and central lines in the emergency department (ED) and the intensive care unit.

Attending physicians are in house to supervise and backup anesthesiology and obstetric (OB) residents and collaborate with CRNAs in the delivery of anesthesia services. No midwives are on the OB service hospital staff, and no doulas are employed by the hospital.

There are 20 labor-delivery rooms where women labor and deliver their babies. Two C-Section rooms are available for operative deliveries. A level 2 neonatal care unit and neonatal nursery are in the childbirth unit.

Equipment and monitoring in patient rooms include oxygen, suction, and electronic monitoring (EFM) for patient and baby and two transportable monitors on wheels. Both C-section rooms have EFM that can be moved. Transportable vital sign and pulse oximetry monitors are available from other patient floors. Nitrous oxide is available for labor analgesia by portable tank system and is provided/monitored by a labor and delivery nurse. Postpartum patients can be relocated to patient rooms of a post-surgery care unit down the hallway from the childbirth unit until discharge to open childbirth beds. A recent influx of OB patients caused the hospital to expand bed space to the hallways. This stretched the nurse-to-staff ratio and monitoring equipment availability.

Professional interpreter services are available in the hospital but poorly staffed on the weekends. In the past, Spanish-speaking housekeeping personnel have assisted in interpretation. Three childbirth unit nurses speak Spanish, but only one is assigned to work this weekend. Patient family members have also been used to interpret to inform and obtain consent for general care and necessary procedures. Some unit nurses have employed language interpretation software via their cellphones to communicate with non-English-speaking patients (Elred, 2008; Youdelman, 2019).

The charge nurse has notified you that an 18-year-old Spanish-speaking patient in latent labor has just been admitted to the childbirth unit. Due to a lack of bed space, the patient is placed on a gurney in the hallway adjoining the nurses' station. The admitting obstetrician-gynecologist (OB/GYN) has ordered an IV followed by placement of an epidural for labor and delivery analgesia (Aderemi, 2016; American College of Obstetricians & Gynecologists, 2017; Torres & De Vries, 2009). You are currently engaged with the placement of a continuous epidural for labor and delivery in the childbirth unit. It may take 45 to 60 minutes before you are available to assess the newly admitted latent labor patient currently located in the childbirth unit hallway (American College of Obstetricians & Gynecologists, 2019; Apfelbaum et al., 2016).

The 18-year-old patient, Dolores, is Gravida 1, Para 0 (G1P0) at 38 weeks, but the baby seems small for gestational age. A physical and vaginal exam performed in the ED showed cervical dilation is 2 to 3 cm with membranes intact. Fetal heart rate is regular as per ultrasound. Ultrasound showed a baby in cephalic posterior position but not engaged. Laboratory results and blood cross-match are pending. Dolores is breathing with her contractions. Diagnosis is latent labor. She has been admitted to the childbirth unit for antenatal care. No IV has yet been placed (Beck et al., 2019; Gimovsky et al., 2017; Hui et al., 2010).

Dolores did not have prenatal care (Belasco, n.d.; Health Resources & Services Administration, Maternal and Child Health, n.d.). She has been living with her cousin's family for the last year after immigrating from Honduras. She works in environmental/housekeeping services at a local hotel. Her cousin accompanied her to the hospital ED. Dolores does not have medical insurance. The ED reports that pain management for Dolores was discussed with her cousin present, and Dolores is reported to have said, "Well, I've never felt it, but I imagine pain is just part of the process, and I was told by the women in my family that birth pain is part of giving life. Besides, my cousin said she knows women who have backaches from the epidural. If my baby is in trouble, then maybe I can have it placed, but I will ask the doctor" (Gonzalez et al., 2021; Orejuela et al., 2012; University of Virginia, 2014).

With your knowledge of obstetrics anesthesia and its consequence, how would/could you respond?

Consider:

1. Identify the ethical concerns with this situation.

2. What information will you need before a responsible decision can be made? (Consider what the information is and where it will come from.)

3. Who are stakeholders involved in the decision, and what is the process in which those involved could come to a decision (e.g., what tools are/could be used to create an informed decision)?

4. What are the values relevant to this problem? *Values* are the things that you believe are important in making the decision. They (should) determine priorities. Values relevant to this problem may not be representative of your own personal values or moral framework.

5. What are the options for the decision? Think in terms of values and feasibility (e.g., financial, political, organizational, religious constraints).

Management of Case Study

After all considerations, write a short narrative of how you believe is the best way to manage this situation; list core values important to you for managing the situation.

References

Aderemi, R. A. (2016). Ethical issues in maternal and child health nursing: Challenges faced by maternal and child health nurses and strategies for decision making. *International Journal of Medicine and Biomedical Research*, *5*(2), 67–76. https://www.ajol.info/index.php/ijmbr/article/view/142404

American College of Obstetricians and Gynecologists. (2017). ACOG Practice Bulletin No. 177: Obstetric analgesia and anesthesia. *Obstetrics & Gynecology*, *129*(4), e73–e89. https://doi.org/10.1097/AOG.0000000000002018

American College of Obstetricians and Gynecologists. (2019). ACOG Committee Opinion No. 766: Approaches to limit intervention during labor and birth. *Obstetrics and Gynecology*, *133*(2), e164–e173. https://doi.org/10.1097/AOG.0000000000003074

Apfelbaum, J. L., Hawkins, J. L., Agarkar, M., Bucklin, B. A., Connis, R. T., Gambling, D. R., Mhyre, J., Nickinovich, D. G., Sherman, H., Tsen, L. C., & Yaghmour, E. T. (2016). Practice guidelines for obstetric anesthesia: An updated report by the American Society of Anesthesiologists Task Force on Obstetric Anesthesia and the Society for Obstetric Anesthesia and Perinatology. *Anesthesiology, 124*(2), 270–300.

Beck, R., Malvasi, A., Kuczkowski, K. M., Marinelli, E., & Zaami, S. (2019). Intrapartum sonography of fetal head in second stage of labor with neuraxial analgesia: A literature review and possible medicolegal aftermath. *European Review for Medical and Pharmacological Sciences, 23*(8), 3159–3166. https://doi.org/10.26355/eurrev_201904_17673

Belasco, J. (n.d.). *Behind from the start: Why some women aren't receiving early prenatal care — Part 2.* USC Annenberg, Center for Health Journalism, Fellowship Story Showcase. https://centerforhealthjournalism.org/fellowships/projects/behind-start-why-some-women-arent-receiving-early-prenatal-care

Elred, S. M. (2008, August 15). *With scarce access to interpreters, immigrants struggle to understand doctors' orders.* NPR. https://www.npr.org/sections/health-shots/2018/08/15/638913165/with-scarce-access-to-medical-interpreters-immigrant-patients-struggle-to-understand

Gimovsky, A. C., Guarente, J., & Berghella, V. (2017). Prolonged second stage in nulliparous with epidurals: A systematic review. *Journal of Maternal-Fetal & Neonatal Medicine, 30*(4), 461–465. https://doi.org/10.1080/14767058.2016.1174999

Gonzalez, B., Gonzalez, S. R., Rojo, M., & Mhyre, J. (2021). Neuraxial analgesia in pregnant Hispanic women: An assessment of their beliefs and expectations. *International Journal of Women's Health, 13,* 87–94. https://doi.org/10.2147/IJWH.S270711

Health Resources & Services Administration, Maternal and Child Health. (n.d.). *Healthy start.* https://mchb.hrsa.gov/programs-impact/healthy-start

Hui, J., Hahn, P. M., Jamieson, M. A., & Palerme, S. (2010). The duration of labor in adolescents. *Journal of Pediatric and Adolescent Gynecology, 23*(4), 226–229. https://doi.org/10.1016/j.jpag.2010.01.001

Orejuela, F. J., Garcia, T., Green, C., Kilpatrick, C., Guzman, S., & Blackwell, S. (2012). Exploring factors influencing patient request for epidural analgesia on admission to labor and delivery in a predominantly Latino population. *Journal of Immigrant and Minority Health, 14*(2), 287–291.

Torres, J. M., & De Vries, R. G. (2009). Birthing ethics: What mothers, families, childbirth educators, nurses, and physicians should know about the ethics of childbirth. *The Journal of Perinatal Education, 18*(1), 12–24.

University of Virginia. (2014, February 4). Hispanic women opt for labor pain relief less often than others. *ScienceDaily.* https://www.sciencedaily.com/releases/2014/02/140204101414.htm

Youdelman, M. (2019, April 29). Summary of state law requirements addressing language needs in health care. *National Health Law Program.* https://healthlaw.org/resource/summary-of-state-law-requirements-addressing-language-needs-in-health-care-2/

VIOLENCE, SUICIDE, AND FAMILY DYNAMICS WITH MEDICAL COMPLEXITY

When caring for patients, advanced practice registered nurses (APRNs) are often faced with conflicting information without having a means to verify the accuracy of what they are being told. While this type of scenario is always challenging, it becomes distressing to providers when the concerns being voiced are germane to not only the safety of the patient but also others in the community. APRNs are increasingly being tasked with assessing individuals for the risk for not only suicide but also violence toward others. While this often falls in the purview of psychiatric mental health nurse practitioners (PMHNPs), any APRN may find themselves in the situation where they need to do an initial assessment and determine next steps. Suicidal behaviors and violence are complex phenomena with a plethora of distal and proximal risk factors (Ryan & Oquendo, 2020; Skeem & Monahan, 2011). It is important to remember that assessment does not equal prediction. Just as it is impossible to predict the weather with 100% certainty, it is impossible to predict whether a person will go on to die by suicide (Ryan & Oquendo, 2020). Predictions surrounding violence toward others are equally as challenging.

Assessment allows APRNs to use the information they have about an individual regarding their risk and protective factors for suicide, along with their warning signs and behaviors to mitigate as many of those risks as possible, while also promoting safety, health, and resiliency to decrease the likelihood that they will go on to die by suicide (Ryan & Oquendo, 2020). Violence risk assessments are similar because many of the underlying risk and protective factors, as well as warning signs and behaviors, are similar. There are no biomarkers, imaging studies, or laboratory findings that can tell a healthcare professional whether a person is likely to kill themselves (Ryan & Oquendo, 2020) or another. Suicide and violence risk assessments are inherently challenging in that providers are charged with the daunting task of obtaining a tremendous amount of information from a patient in a sensitive manner about their personality, coping skills, resiliency, stressors, behaviors, emotional states, and current thinking; compare that with what they are observing and being told by others; and condense it all into a risk assessment to determine whether there is a high likelihood of the patient killing themselves or bringing harm to another person in the near future. Once risk is identified, the provider is then tasked with determining the next steps to mitigate the identified risk and attempt to ensure safety.

The laws governing actions taken by providers after a person is deemed to be at "imminent" risk to self or others vary greatly throughout the country (Treatment Advocacy Center, 2018). Each state has a mechanism to detain a person for a brief time period to ensure they are assessed, with additional mechanisms to allow longer periods of detention and potentially treatment based upon that initial assessment. However, the laws vary greatly in terms of their time frames for the initial detention of the patient, where the detention occurs, whether treatment may be provided against a patient's will, and what steps must be taken to protect a patient's civil rights (Treatment Advocacy Center, 2018). The laws are often not clear in defining what presents "dangerousness" and what time frame of said dangerousness warrants detention or commitment (Testa & West, 2010). This can lead even providers who work with the laws regularly to be confused and frustrated. Family members and other healthcare providers less familiar with these laws are frequently frustrated and frightened when they believe that an individual is dangerous and not enough is being done to maintain safety. If there is a bad outcome, such as a patient dying by suicide or harming another, the provider often is blamed for not assessing the patient well enough or predicting that the action would occur. This leads to performing suicide and violence risk assessments in an environment with a fear of liability and perceived responsibility, which has the potential to result in treatment and interventions that are more restrictive than necessary and potentially harmful and traumatic to patients (Ryan & Oquendo, 2020).

In addition to practicing within all applicable state laws regarding the need to potentially detain a patient due to them presenting an imminent danger to themselves or others, all providers have an ethical and legal obligation to maintain confidentiality regarding what patients disclose to them as part of their treatment. However, if that patient represents a danger to others, and sometimes even themselves, the provider may have an obligation to warn others regarding the patient and violate their privacy. Like determining which actions to take regarding involuntary detention and treatment, the legal requirements vary from state to state regarding "duty to warn" and "duty to protect" when a patient is deemed to be dangerous (National Conference of State Legislatures, 2022).

Some states have mandatory duty to warn and duty to protect laws, whereas in others the laws are permissive and disclosure is not required, but if a provider believes there is a "clear and immediate danger to others or to society," confidentiality may be breached, and the information may be reported (National Conference of State Legislatures, 2022, para. 4). These laws protect providers from liability when they are breaching confidentiality in good faith (National Conference of State Legislatures, 2022). There are states that have no duty to warn or protect laws, and others where the responsibilities differ depending on the profession. Again, the varying patchwork of laws with unclear definitions often leads to reticence and fear among providers who do not face these situations regularly. They may find themselves asking: Is the danger "immediate enough" to detain this person against their will? If I do detain them, does that do any good, and can

I treat them if they are detained? If I can't detain them any longer and I am releasing them, if I warn law enforcement or their family, am I doing them more harm or will I violate HIPAA? Will they sue me?

These scenarios are even more challenging when you as a provider are being told different stories by the patient and their family and don't have a good way to verify anything you are being told or know who to believe. You want to do the right thing and protect your patient and the community, but how do you know what is accurate?

Violence, Suicide, and Family Dynamics Case Study

Peter is a 68-year-old male with a past medical history of recurrent metastatic prostate cancer, depression, and anxiety (both diagnoses in context of cancer recurrence) who was brought to the emergency department (ED) by police after recurrent calls to emergency services by his daughter and son-in-law for increasingly erratic behavior that culminated in him saying he would kill himself via carbon monoxide poisoning, going to his garage, and attempting to get into his car and turn it on. In the ED, he was alert and oriented to self, date, location, and situation. He was cooperative with care, appeared to be in no apparent distress, told the ED physician that he still wanted to kill himself as he was "sick of it all," and said that if she left him alone for 10 minutes, he'd figure out how to do it. He was seen by social work (SW), to whom he made similar statements.

In addition to speaking with Peter, SW spoke with his daughter. She had moved from out of state about two months prior to move in with Peter and his wife to help care for them as they had learned that Peter's cancer was terminal. The daughter reported that Peter has had significant behavior changes over the past two to three months, including increased irritability and being emotionally, physically, and sexually abusive toward his wife. His behavior had become so extreme toward his wife that she had started the process for separation and moved out of their home during the previous month. The daughter reported that she and her husband, who moved with her to care for them, no longer felt safe in the home with her dad because of his behavior. She described how he has ignited his wife's belongings that remain in the home. In fact, the morning that he was brought to the hospital, the daughter had awoken to the smell of smoke and found him burning items on the living room floor.

Based upon the statements made by Peter to the ED attending and the collateral information provided by his daughter and the police officers who brought him to the hospital, the ED SW placed him on an involuntary psychiatric hold and referred him for admission to geriatric psychiatry. Peter began boarding in the ED while awaiting an inpatient bed because there was not one readily available. Initially, in the ED, no lab work or head imaging had been done because he had been seen at his oncologist's office recently, and those labs were reviewed and found to be unremarkable. He was started on his home medications, which included duloxetine 30mg daily and buspirone 7.5mg twice daily.

The following morning, Peter mentioned not being able to eat for several days due to mouth sores, which he attributed to the new palliative chemotherapy agent that was started two weeks prior. He complained of dizziness and appeared unsteady on his feet. Orthostatic vital signs were obtained, and he was found to be hypotensive at baseline with a significant drop in blood pressure upon standing. A complete blood count, comprehensive metabolic panel, and urinalysis (UA) were then obtained. His labs were significant for leukocytosis, anemia, thrombocytopenia, and hypernatremia. His UA was without evidence of infection. He remained afebrile and later became mildly tachycardic. Due to his leukocytosis and persistent hypotension with significant orthostasis, he met criteria for systemic inflammatory response syndrome with concern for sepsis. Therefore, the plan was switched to admit him to a medical unit with a psychiatric consultation. Blood cultures were obtained, and he was started on intravenous fluids. As Peter was on a psychiatric hold, he required a one-to-one observer for admission; therefore, he continued to board in the psychiatric area of the ED while awaiting a medical bed and the staff for a one to one. While boarding in the ED, his care transitioned to the inpatient medicine service. A psychiatric consultation was requested.

17

You are the PMHNP working on the Psychiatric Consult-Liaison Service. Peter's consultation was assigned to you and the PMHNP student you are precepting. You see him in the ED on his first day of boarding after spending one night in the ED. Your student conducts most of the psychiatric assessment while you observe and ask additional questions as necessary. You find Peter walking around the psychiatric area of the ED with a front wheel walker, talking with staff and asking when he can "get the hell out of here."

Peter is quite happy to meet with you as he believes that you will help him get out of the hospital. He shows you to his room in the ED, leaves his walker there, and walks back out to the hallway to grab an additional chair for the student. He declines your offer to get the chair or to assist him. He is well kempt in hospital pajamas, overly friendly and talkative with somewhat pressured, loud speech. He is hard of hearing and requires many questions to be repeated. He relays the events leading up to his admission regarding how he wanted to kill himself and went to the garage and tried to start the car to use carbon monoxide. Peter says it was all a huge mistake and he regrets it because it "landed me here." He denies wanting to kill himself and discusses his impending death, being told he has three months to live and being "all black inside from the cancer."

When questioned about symptoms of depression and anxiety, Peter denies symptoms consistent with a major depressive disorder or an anxiety disorder. He acknowledges distress, emotional pain, and fear related to his terminal diagnosis and his wife leaving him. Peter describes that he wanted to kill himself the day prior because he "had just had it with his daughter, son-in-law, and their huge dog." He spoke about the lack of control and freedom he felt in his own home with them there and not knowing what to do. He acknowledged saying hurtful things to them and his wife but denied physically threatening or harming anyone and said, "Who told you that?" Peter denied access to firearms, stated his "daughter and son-in-law brought a bunch with them when they moved in," but reported they were all stored in a locker, and he didn't know how to open it. Peter went on to spontaneously talk about how he doesn't like guns and didn't see the need for them. He denied any psychotic symptoms, including audio and visual hallucinations.

You noted no evidence of delusions or obsessions throughout the assessment. He was oriented to self and hospital but unsure of day and month. He correctly stated the year. He appeared to be confused and confabulating at times. He spoke about what was on the hospital property before it was built and mentioned building the hospital. He acknowledged short-term memory issues and word finding problems, which he estimates he has had for two weeks or so. Bedside cognitive and attentional testing revealed significant deficits in attention and executive functioning, which would impact impulse control and problem-solving and could be suggestive of organic etiologies such as metastases or delirium, especially as family had reported a rather abrupt change in behavior. Peter agreed to imaging of his head to rule out metastases to the brain. He also gave permission to call his daughter and gather more information.

The PMHNP student called his daughter and spoke with her at length. She confirmed the information she had previously told ED SW and provided additional information. She confirmed that she had observed some word finding issues and forgetfulness in the last "couple of weeks" and described that her father has always been irritable and had a temper but that his behavior beginning two months ago represents an abrupt change. She reported that over 30 years ago when he was a heavy drinker, he had been physically abusive to his wife, herself, and her siblings, but after getting sober, the physical abuse stopped. She denied any past psychiatric history, treatment, or suicidal behaviors. She confirmed that he had no access to firearms. She agreed with additional workup to rule out metastases to the brain.

In reviewing his outpatient records, you note that Peter was diagnosed with anxiety and depression in the context of his third recurrence of metastatic prostate cancer. His Patient Health Questionnaire–9 and General Anxiety Disorder–7 scale scores were erratic, often inconsistent with the narrative he reported to his doctor, and improved or worsened from visit to visit without any intervention. He consistently declined referral to counseling or mental health services. He was started on duloxetine once, took it for a few days, then called his doctor and told them it made him "nuttier than a bed bug," and he refused to take it anymore. Later he was started on buspirone 5mg twice daily, which he appeared to take regularly. He had been restarted on duloxetine three months prior to admission by palliative care for pain, and the buspirone was increased after he was given his terminal diagnosis.

As Peter is being worked up for sepsis with a white count that continues to climb, it is inappropriate to diagnosis him with any psychiatric disorders because medical etiologies for behavioral and psychological symptoms must be ruled out first. However, based upon his age, lack of prior psychiatric history, lack of symptoms consistent with a major depressive disorder or anxiety disorder, and abrupt onset of behavioral symptoms that appear to be worsening, along with what appear to be new onset cognitive deficits in the context of metastatic cancer along with numerous psychosocial stressors, you find it highly unlikely that his symptoms are related to an underlying psychiatric disorder. You also doubt that inpatient psychiatry would be of any benefit to him as it is focused on active treatment of psychiatric disorders as opposed to helping a person cope with and prepare for death due to a terminal diagnosis. You maintain the psychiatric hold due to the safety concerns of the family and need for additional workup, and you discontinue the duloxetine due to lack of clear indication and concern for contribution to behavior changes based upon past reports of adverse effects. You recommend an MRI with and without contrast of the brain to rule out metastases and discuss your recommendations with the internist, who agrees to order the MRI.

The following day when you see Peter, he continues to deny thoughts of suicide, expresses remorse for his behavior, makes statements regarding his daughter and son-in-law lying about him so "you'll keep me here," and talks about them trying to take his property and money. He continues to have erratic BP and HR, with intermittent tachycardia up to the 140s at times, and hypotension. He remains disoriented to time and continues to confabulate. His MRI showed no evidence of metastases. You are concerned about the potential for autoimmune paraneoplastic encephalitis based upon his metastatic disease and lack of other clear etiology for abrupt behavioral and cognitive changes. However, the yield of the workup for autoimmune paraneoplastic encephalitis that includes a lumbar puncture with cerebrospinal fluid studies, which can take up to two weeks to return in a terminal patient with cancer that cannot be excised or treated, appears to be quite low. You recommend a neurology consultation. Peter's oncologist had been in touch with the teaching service and agreed with consideration of autoimmune paraneoplastic encephalitis, though he felt it was unlikely. He believes Peter's symptoms are caused by post-traumatic stress disorder (PTSD) and wanted to know why treatment was not being initiated for that. The oncologist also felt that his leukocytosis was related to his chemotherapy and not an infection. His blood cultures returned negative that evening.

Peter was seen by neurology the following day; at that time, he was fully oriented and displayed no attentional or memory deficits. Neurology did not feel there would be a benefit from additional workup. You see Peter later that day, and his cognition and memory were indeed greatly improved from when you'd seen him previously. The county mental health investigator concluded her investigation and did not believe that civil commitment was warranted. Therefore, Peter could only be detained in the hospital for a short time longer until a safe plan for discharge could be worked out. Based upon his improvement in symptomatology and lack of psychiatric symptoms, you agreed with this plan, asked the social worker to start working on safety planning, and removed Peter from the list for inpatient psychiatry. His oral intake had improved, and he was eating three meals a day and drinking plenty of fluids. He remained mildly tachycardic, but his hypotension had improved, and he was no longer reporting dizziness.

Upon learning that Peter would not be civilly committed and could not be detained in the hospital for much longer, his daughter called the primary team, spoke with the intern, and voiced concern that if discharged he would kill his wife, his other daughter, and potentially her. She was insisting that he not be discharged and that it was unsafe to do so. The following morning, you learn of these statements from the primary team as they are all very concerned and frightened regarding discharge. They do not understand why you won't just admit him to psychiatry, questioning why this is not PTSD as the oncologist "who knows him much better believes" and asking "How can we discharge such a dangerous person?"

You explain why Peter's symptoms are inconsistent with a primary psychiatric disorder, that based on what his family is reporting he may have a personality disorder, and that at this point, he has been completely cooperative and has not displayed any of the behaviors they say he has throughout his hospital stay. At this point there is no legal recourse to detain him further in the hospital unless he lacks capacity to make his own decisions, and there is no safe place to discharge him to, neither of which appear to be accurate. When safe discharge was brought up, the team mentions that the daughter has stated that Peter is unable to manage his finances or cook. This is new information. You feel pressured to start antipsychotic medication to make him less irritable and an antidepressant for his assumed PTSD. You explain that his current symptoms do not warrant the medications, and the benefits do not outweigh the risks. Due to their ongoing discomfort, you do agree to call the daughter as it is unknown if the wife has begun to pursue a restraining order and to clarify these new concerns regarding finances and cooking.

When you call the daughter, you note that she seems to be telling you different information than she told your PMHNP student when collateral information was initially gathered. She is now describing more violent and threatening behavior than previously; you discuss restraining orders with her. She reports that her mother and sister are in the process of getting one. She then goes on to say, "But that won't stop him from getting a gun from someone else." The daughter mentions Peter having numerous firearms, so you discuss with her options to remove the firearms while Peter is in the hospital and note that if a restraining order is granted, he will be restricted from purchasing additional firearms. She then says, "He'll just get one from a friend." You explain how Peter will be educated by the deputies who serve him with a restraining order regarding the risk of such action. She then starts talking about him taking one of the many cars they have and finding his wife even though he doesn't know where she is. You suggest to her that his wife ensure that she removes all the car keys prior to his discharge as part of her safety planning, as they are also her property. The daughter then says that will work until he gets the car re-keyed.

Next, she moved on to talking about all the reasons Peter would be unsafe at home alone. She reports he can't cook, can't go shopping, and doesn't know how to manage finances or take his medications. You ask her when he began having difficulty with those tasks, and she says, "He's never known how to do them, mom always did all that. He can't even make a cup of coffee." She states that he has kicked her out of the house, so she and her husband are planning to leave because they don't feel safe anyway, so there will be no one to help him when he gets home. You explain that if she doesn't feel safe and he has told her to leave that is for the better. You thank her for notifying you of the concerns regarding meals, medications, and finances so that a safe solution can be worked out prior to his discharge, as the patient will no longer have their support at home. She then asks you what you are going to do to ensure all the animals are taken care of and mentions there are a variety of animals on the property (chickens, goats, dogs) and that her father is unable to care for them. You advise her that if she is sure he can't care for them then she should call the Humane Society. You then end the phone call, as it has become clear that her focus seems to be on ensuring that her father remains in the hospital, and additional problems are brought up with every solution offered.

When seeing Peter that afternoon, you take SW with you to continue working on discharge planning. Much of the conversation centers around how Peter will take care of himself. He expresses feeling quite relieved knowing his daughter and son-in-law are moving out and that he can finally sleep well. You talk with him about how he will manage without any help and specifically mention cooking. Peter states, "I can cook just fine, I've done it my whole life." You ask him about his favorite meal to cook, and he is able to describe step by step how to prepare it and make adjustments as needed based on available ingredients. Peter is also able to describe his finances and problem solve some of the work around his home, including animal care and other issues. He expresses concern over how his other daughter is treating his wife but has no desire to go and find her; instead, he says he'll go talk to a lawyer about it when he gets out of the hospital to make sure she has everything she needs. The description his daughter provided of his abilities does not match what he seems capable of based upon your assessment. After you leave, Peter continues to talk with SW and mentions that he found it odd that he feels so much better since being in the hospital and wonders if his daughter was doing something funny with his medications when she gave them to him. He also mentions that she only fed him one meal a day. Later you realize that what the daughter told you about guns was very different from what she had told your student initially and did not match what the patient reported upon admission.

Consider:

1. Identify the ethical concerns with this situation.

2. What information will you need before a responsible decision can be made? (Consider what the information is and where it will come from.)

3. Who are stakeholders involved in the decision, and what is the process in which those involved could come to a decision (e.g., what tools are/could be used to create an informed decision)?

4. What are the values relevant to this problem? *Values* are the things that you believe are important in making the decision. They (should) determine priorities. Values relevant to this problem may not be representative of your own personal values or moral framework.

5. What are the options for the decision? Think in terms of values and feasibility (e.g., financial, political, organizational, religious constraints).

Management of Case Study

After all considerations, write a short narrative of how you believe is the best way to manage this situation; list core values important to you for managing the situation.

References

National Conference of State Legislatures. (2022). *Mental health professionals' duty to warn.* https://www.ncsl.org/research/health/mental-health-professionals-duty-to-warn.aspx

Ryan, E. P., & Oquendo, M. A. (2020). Suicide risk assessment and prevention: Challenges and opportunities. *FOCUS, 18*(2), 88–99. https://doi.org/10.1176/appi.focus.20200011

Skeem, J. L., & Monahan, J. (2011). Current directions in violence risk assessment. *Current Directions in Psychological Science, 20*(1), 38–42. https://doi.org/10.1177/0963721410397271

Testa, M., & West, S. (2010). Civil commitment in the United States. *Psychiatry, 7*(10), 30–40.

Treatment Advocacy Center. (2018). *State treatment laws.* https://www.treatmentadvocacycenter.org/fixing-the-system/state-treatment-laws

DELIRIUM AND FALL RISK IN ACUTE CARE

Falls and violence are significant safety issues in acute care hospitals. Falls account for the largest number of reported adverse events in hospitals and are considered the most serious safety issue for hospitalized elderly patients (Hicks, 2015; Moore & Geist, 2015). Patient falls during admissions result in harm to patients and an increased burden to individuals and the healthcare system via injuries, deaths, increased length of stay, and greater than $41,570 in additional charges per hospitalization (Inouye et al., 2009; Peterson et al., 2021). Patient violence is a leading cause of healthcare worker injury, illness, and days away from work, with rates of violence increasing throughout the United States (Derscheid et al., 2021). Falls and violence are both considered preventable through the application of evidence-based interventions that focus on identifying risk and initiating appropriate interventions based upon the identified risk level (Derscheid et al., 2021; Ghosh et al., 2019; Hicks, 2015; Moore & Geist, 2015; Rowan & Veenema, 2017). Bedside nursing staff often bear the brunt of activities aimed at risk assessment and initiating care plans with individualized interventions based upon the identified risk.

Although there are numerous validated falls and violence risk assessment tools, they lack validity when applied broadly throughout an acute care hospital due to the complexity of each issue (Derscheid et al., 2021; Ghosh et al., 2019; Rowan & Veenema, 2017). Falls and violence are often patient safety issues that were present long before a patient ever arrives at the hospital; staff then become tasked with preventing an often long-standing issue during treatment for an acute illness and feeling responsible if these events occur due to the focus placed on prevention. Delirium is the most common neuropsychiatric syndrome encountered in the acute care setting, though it is often unrecognized (Maldonado, 2017). Along with increasing morbidity and mortality, delirium increases the risk for falls and episodes of violence during hospitalization (Derscheid et al., 2021; Maldonado, 2017; Sillner et al., 2019). The interventions aimed at reducing falls (limited mobility) and violence (psychotropic medications) often increase the likelihood that a patient will develop delirium, thus further increasing their risk for falls and violence.

In 2002, the National Quality Forum listed "patient death or serious disability associated with a fall while being cared for in a healthcare facility" to its list of "Never Events" (Lembitz & Clarke, 2009). This was followed in 2008 by the Centers for Medicare & Medicaid Services' (CMS) subsequent adoption of the non-reimbursement policy for a subset of these "never events" that included falls (Inouye et al., 2009; Lembitz & Clarke, 2009). The goal for considering falls "never" and "no pay" events was to reduce their occurrence in healthcare due to the burden they add to individual patients and to the healthcare system. At the time, the authors of the CMS rule acknowledged there was no evidence that falls "can be consistently and effectively prevented through the application of evidence-based guidelines" (Inouye et al., 2009, p. 239).

While reducing falls in healthcare is an important goal, the placement of falls on the list equating them to preventable medical errors—such as wrong site surgery—appears to have been an aspirational means to incentivize healthcare systems to make systemic change to improve care but without available evidence of efficacy while also investing in additional research on the topic. Since that time, systems have allocated significant resources to falls prevention through quality improvement and research (Hicks, 2015; Inouye et al., 2009; Rowan & Veenema, 2017). Concern is frequently raised by bedside providers and caregivers, as well as in the literature, that the focus on fall prevention with a goal of no falls has unintended consequences of furthering patient harm through the restriction of mobility, application of mechanical restraints, and reallocation of resources from other areas that could have a greater impact on patient safety (Inouye et al., 2009; Lembitz & Clarke, 2009). Some interventions frequently used to prevent falls such as net-enclosure beds have little evidence to support their efficacy or evaluate their negative effects (Haynes & Pratt, 2009; Nawaz et al., 2007).

Psychiatric Acute Concerns and Fall Risks Case Study

Marilyn is an 82-year-old widowed woman with a past medical history significant for hypertension, breast cancer status post double mastectomy and radiation treatment in her mid-50s, osteoporosis, and presumed mild cognitive impairment. Her husband died seven years ago, and Marilyn was very active in her community up until the COVID-19 pandemic. She volunteered regularly at the local senior center, was active in church and Rotary club, golfed and swam regularly, and walked daily for exercise. During the pandemic, she followed guidelines for quarantine and social isolation stringently and stopped her activities. Unfortunately, her daughter moved out of town a few months prior to the beginning of the pandemic, leading to further isolation. Her other two adult children also live out of town. Throughout the pandemic, Marilyn has ordered her groceries online and done all other shopping online. She has attended church services online and maintained regular contact with her children and grandchildren via video calls. She continued walking outdoors regularly but stopped all her other typical activities, including driving.

18

Marilyn's daughter came to visit after being called by one of her neighbors, who notified her that Marilyn had failed to pay the homeowner's association dues for multiple months despite having reminders sent and that her yard was in disarray. When Marilyn's daughter arrived, she found the house to be less tidy than typical, with multiple piles of unopened mail including unpaid bills. She realized her mother hadn't gone to any medical appointments for the last two years and that she seemed to be having difficulties with her memory. She learned that Marilyn had fallen a few times in her home and once while on one of her outdoor walks. Her falls seemed to be associated with tripping, such as over uneven surfaces or her clothing. One night during her daughter's visit, Marilyn fell while getting up to go to the bathroom and hit her head. She had tripped over the bathmat on the bathroom floor. Her daughter took her to the local emergency department (ED). Her head computed tomography (CT) scan showed no acute intracranial abnormalities and generalized atrophy commensurate with her age, and her vital signs (VS) were stable. No lab work was done. As her daughter had reported that Marilyn tends to have difficulty sleeping and is "restless" in the evening, Marilyn was started on a low dose of quetiapine, 12.5mg nightly, in the ED. Marilyn's daughter was able to extend her visit and helped her mother get her financial affairs back in order and follow up with her primary care provider (PCP) for a routine checkup. With the support of her children and her PCP, Marilyn made the difficult decision to move into an assisted living facility (ALF) nearby. She felt good about the decision, as many of her friends from church had moved there over the last decade or so and had nice things to say about it. Her children sold her home and vehicle.

Five weeks after moving into the ALF, Marilyn was brought to the ED due to increased agitation in her facility. Over the previous week, she had become increasingly disruptive with decreased sleep, walking into other residents' rooms without invitation, becoming verbally assaultive when redirected, and hitting and kicking at staff. She also left the facility twice stating she was "done visiting and was going back home." Both times staff were able to follow and convince her to return rather reluctantly. The events that led to the facility calling 911 and requesting transport to the ED involved Marilyn slapping another resident when they told her not to come into their room. The staff at the ALF are requesting admission to geriatric psychiatry for management of Marilyn's behavioral dyscontrol.

In the ED, Marilyn presents as confused though alert and oriented to self, day, date, and hospital. She was somewhat irritable, requesting to go home and not understanding why she had been brought there. She denied that she hit anyone and stated she would never do such a thing. Her VS were stable with temperature of 97.9, blood pressure of 92/64, heart rate of 96, respiratory rate of 18, and oxygen saturation of 97% on room air. Repeat head imaging was not done as there were no reported concerns of additional falls from her facility. Complete blood count (CBC) showed mild anemia, and comprehensive metabolic panel (CMP) showed mild hypernatremia and mild hyperkalemia. Creatinine increased to 1.08mg/dL from her baseline average of 0.9mg/dL, albumin of 2.8g/dL, and eGFR of 51mL/min/1.73m2. The staff at her facility were unable to provide information regarding her recent food and fluid intake.

The ED attending requested a social work (SW) evaluation in ED as Marilyn's facility had requested geriatric psychiatry admission prior to accepting her back. SW met with Marilyn briefly and did not feel that referral to geriatric psychiatry was warranted based upon her current symptomatology because she has no history of any psychiatric disorder, and her behavior change appears related to potential neurocognitive impairment or a medical etiology compounded by her recent move. A urine sample was not obtained as Marilyn did not urinate while in ED. She received a liter of intravenous (IV) fluids and was admitted to a medical floor under observation status for further workup and disposition planning. She was continued on her home medications, hydrochlorothiazide 12.5mg daily and quetiapine 25mg twice daily. At some point, the quetiapine that had been started during her previous ED visit when she fell had been increased to 25mg twice daily. A psychiatry consultation was ordered to assist in placement at the request of care management. Additionally, Marilyn had become quite agitated on the first night of her admission, attempting to elope from the hospital to "go back home." Marilyn tripped and fell while

18

trying to evade staff to get out of the hospital. She did not hit her head; however, she did incur a mild abrasion on one knee.

When staff tried to assist her back to her room, she reportedly became combative, hitting, kicking, and biting at nurses. She was given olanzapine 5mg via intramuscular injection (IM) and required mechanical restraints due to her behavior. Within 30 minutes of olanzapine IM and mechanical restraint, she fell asleep, and the restraints were removed. However, six hours later when she woke, she was again agitated, demanding to leave and trying to get out of bed. She was given an additional 5mg of oral olanzapine due to her agitation and behavioral dyscontrol. The IM and oral olanzapine as well as the mechanical restraints were ordered by the hospitalist providing overnight cross coverage who was unfamiliar with her case. The nursing staff placed a one to one (1:1) with Marilyn after she woke up agitated to reassure her, help keep her calm, prevent elopement, and provide redirection and de-escalation to prevent the need for further as needed (prn) medication and mechanical restraint.

You are the psychiatric mental health nurse practitioner (PMHNP) working on the psychiatric consult-liaison service who received the consultation request for Marilyn. The consultation question from the primary team in the order was, "Please assess for gero psych and adjust medications due to ongoing agitation." Prior to seeing Marilyn, you talk to the family nurse practitioner (FNP) who is the attending nurse for Marilyn and review the electronic medical record (EMR). Her records prior to moving into the ALF are available through your hospital's EMR. You do not see any cognitive testing done previously that would provide the basis for the diagnosis of "presumed mild cognitive impairment." Additionally, it appears that Marilyn has lost 17 pounds in the last two years, representing a 12% reduction in her weight. You note that the quetiapine was increased in the last two weeks as the facility had called her PCP reporting increased agitation. Marilyn's medication adherence at her facility is unclear, as a medication administration record was not sent with her. Overnight, nursing staff were able to obtain a urine sample from Marilyn; her urinalysis results are consistent with a urinary tract infection (UTI) with culture pending. She was started on IV antibiotics by the primary team.

Upon examination, you find Marilyn sleeping soundly. She is well kempt, in a hospital gown. The certified nursing assistant (CNA), who is her 1:1, reports she's been sleeping all morning and did not wake for breakfast or VS. She doesn't respond to her name being called loudly but does wake when her shoulder is shaken firmly while her name is called. After you raise the head of her bed to keep her in a more seated position, call her name a few more times, and hold her hand while moving it gently, she is more alert. Marilyn agrees to participate in assessment. She is groggy but able to complete the assessment. Marilyn can state her full name, date of birth, and the state in which you are located. Otherwise, she believes it is 30 years prior, and she is unsure of where she is. When given multiple choice options of a hotel, hospital, or supermarket, she accurately states she is in a hospital after looking around her room, though she is unsure why she is there. She denies any past psychiatric history, symptoms of depression or anxiety, lifetime or current suicidal thoughts, and visual and auditory hallu-cinations. She reports that her appetite has been good, denies any concern about weight changes, and denies any alterations in her food/fluid intake. She denies any difficulty with sleep and states that she is a "night owl, always has been" and prefers to sleep late. She denies any pain or discomfort.

Marilyn acknowledges some issues with her memory and that it's dif-ficult to recall names of items and people but denies being concerned about it. She denies that she moved into an ALF recently and states her address as the address of the home she lived at prior to moving. Marilyn showed deficits in her bedside cognitive and attention testing. Though she denied any perceptual disturbances, she did comment on the little children present in the room and pointed at them. There were no children present.

Throughout your assessment, Marilyn is groggy and restless; she attempts to get out of bed multiple times and is easily redirected to stay in bed by distracting her from her goal of getting out of bed. At one point she reports that she needs to use the restroom. You call her nurse into the room to assist as she has IV fluids running and you are worried about her gait due to the amount of olanzapine she received

18

overnight. Marilyn's gait is quite unsteady, and she requires a significant amount of assistance getting up from the bed and ambulating to and from the bathroom from the nurse. Despite feeling as if she had to urinate, she was unable to do so.

After finishing with Marilyn, you call her daughter, who is listed as her medical decision-maker on her advanced directive, to gather additional information. You learn that Marilyn's daughter stayed with her for two weeks after she moved into the ALF to help with the transition and "settle" her in. During that time, she did not notice any behavioral issues with her mother other than the "restless" behavior she had noted previously in the ED when Marilyn presented for falling and hitting her head. She reported that since Marilyn hit her head, she has been a bit more irritable and short-tempered. Her daughter was aware that Marilyn had been having behavioral issues since her departure and that the quetiapine had been increased. She was unsure if Marilyn is taking her medications regularly, as she sometimes refuses them when they are offered because there are more pills than she is accustomed to. Her daughter reports that Marilyn is not the type of person "to just sit around," that she likes to be active, enjoys walking, and even during the pandemic would go on long walks in her neighborhood and the nature reserve nearby. She acknowledged that Marilyn had been falling recently and that the falls were all related to tripping. She stated that in the weeks she was with her mother she observed a steady gait but that Marilyn had difficulty getting up from seated positions and with judging uneven surfaces. The daughter confirmed that Marilyn has no past psychiatric history but she does wonder whether she became "depressed due to the isolation from COVID." She is worried that the ALF won't take her back and reports that she and her siblings aren't sure what to do if they won't, as none of them can move back to town. The daughter also expresses concern regarding the amount of medications her mother has been given and feels like they are making her worse.

You diagnose Marilyn with delirium, mixed state of multifactorial etiology (infectious and metabolic), ruling out neurocognitive disorder as her baseline cognitive status cannot be assessed presently.

You decrease the quetiapine to 12.5mg twice daily with an oral prn of 12.5mg twice daily available for agitation. As you are concerned about larger doses of olanzapine being given, you write an order for 1.25mg IM olanzapine for acute agitation if patient is unable or unwilling to take oral prn medication. You chose to decrease the amount of anti-psychotic medication Marilyn is receiving, as she does not have an underlying psychotic disorder, and it is being used to manage behavioral dyscontrol associated with delirium, superimposed upon a presumed mild cognitive impairment. You realize that while quetiapine and olanzapine can be beneficial in the management of delirium, larger doses may also worsen delirium due to the anticholinergic burden of the two medications. You considered switching to scheduled risperidone from quetiapine; however, as Marilyn had appeared to tolerate low-dose quetiapine well, you elected not to. Melatonin 3mg at dinner is started for sleep/wake cycle restoration and treatment of delirium (Maldonado, 2017).

Additionally, you write a nursing communication order for non-pharmacological delirium interventions that includes keeping blinds open during the day and closed at night, getting patient up to chair with feet on floor as much as possible during the day, reorienting frequently, ambulating in hall at least three times daily with appropriate level of assistance, minimizing night-time interruptions to allow for minimal sleep disruption, working with family to identify familiar topics as well as music and other things she enjoys to incorporate into care, and avoiding centrally acting medications. Lastly, you order vitamin B12, folate, thiamine, and thyroid stimulating hormone (TSH) with reflex free thyroxine labs to evaluate reversible causes of cognitive decline, which was observed prior to the more recent acute change in sensorium and behavior. As Marilyn has lost a significant amount of weight in the last two years, and with her low albumin, you are concerned about malnutrition. You discussed your recommendations with the FNP responsible for Marilyn's care as well as the bedside registered nurse (RN).

The following day, you reviewed Marilyn's chart in the morning. Her TSH, folate, and thiamine were normal. Vitamin B12 level was 158pg/mL, indicating deficiency. She had slept through most of the day after your assessment. Nursing staff were able to wake her for lunch and dinner at which she ate very little. She became "agitated" at approximately 1600, wanting to go home, and she was given a prn of quetiapine, which she readily accepted. She again fell asleep. She could not be woken for her nighttime medications.

At approximately 0100 she became increasingly agitated and confused, wanting to leave. Her nurse attempted to give her a prn of oral quetiapine. She refused it, yelling at the nurse, "You're trying to poison me!" Hospital security had to be called to assist in convincing Marilyn to return to her room. She was described as combative, kicking and hitting at staff, and she received 1.25mg of IM olanzapine. After 15 minutes she remained agitated; the night shift hospitalist was paged and ordered 5mg of haloperidol and 1mg of lorazepam IM. Shortly thereafter Marilyn fell asleep. When you examined her the following morning, Marilyn was sleeping soundly; you were unable to rouse her despite calling her name loudly multiple times and shaking her shoulder. She remained on a 1:1 due to her behavior. The CNA sitting with her in the morning reported she woke up briefly. The CNA was able to get her up to the restroom, where Marilyn had minimal output. She was "very unsteady on her feet." Marilyn then accepted her medications with applesauce from the RN and returned to sleep.

After attempting to wake Marilyn, you speak with the bedside RN. He reports that he is waiting for a net-enclosure bed for Marilyn as she is impulsive and a "huge falls risk;" therefore, one is needed to keep her safe from falls in the hospital as she "doesn't really need a 1:1 because she sleeps most the time," but when she's awake "she's a problem." You review with the bedside RN non-pharmacological delirium interventions and the importance of reorientation, ambulation, cognitive stimulation, and supporting sleep/wake cycle restoration to treat Marilyn's current symptoms, and voice concern that a net-enclosure bed will potentially lead to further behavioral dyscontrol, physical deconditioning, and cognitive decline. He agrees with your concerns and states, "Well, we can't have her fall, and it's not OK for her to be kicking and hitting us. Are you going to increase her meds so she will stop?"

After speaking with the nurse, you speak with the FNP to recommend consideration of B-12 replacement, monitoring intake and output, and minimizing the use of any type of restraints, including net-enclosure beds. The FNP agrees with all recommendations and voices concern about how to manage the nursing staff's request for orders for net-enclosure beds, which must be renewed every 24 hours. You discontinue the haloperidol and lorazepam that were ordered overnight to minimize polypharmacy, write a treatment team "sticky note" in the EMR regarding the importance of minimizing anticholinergic agents and centrally acting drugs, and write a nursing communication order regarding the manufacturer recommendations for net-enclosure beds, which include daily release for ambulation, recreation, nutrition, toileting, and restorative nursing activities.

You next saw Marilyn four days later as it had been a holiday weekend. The PMHNP covering the service had been unable to see her over the weekend due to the volume of new patients. Additionally, Marilyn was transferred to another unit in the hospital to make room for another COVID-19 unit; she is now followed by one of the teaching services. In reviewing her chart, you see that she remains in a net-enclosure bed, the quetiapine has been discontinued, and she is now on scheduled olanzapine 5mg three times daily as it was "more effective." Her urine culture resulted with >100,000 CFUs/mL *Escherichia coli*. IV ciprofloxacin was continued as she was not consistently accepting po medications.

Marilyn continued to have poor oral food and fluid intake. She had also begun retaining urine and is intermittently requiring straight catheterization. Her CBC and basic metabolic panel this morning are consistent with hemoconcentration, though her creatinine has improved to 0.98. IV fluids were restarted this morning.

You find Marilyn sleeping soundly in a net-enclosure bed. She is disheveled, turned around so her head is at the foot of the bed, and the blankets and sheets are all crumpled. You are unable to wake Marilyn despite calling her name multiple times, shaking her shoulder, and doing a sternal rub. She responds to painful stimuli by grunting and shifting position. Her respirations are regular and unlabored. You

18

speak with her bedside nurse regarding your concerns about the on-going use of the net-enclosure bed. Her nurse voiced concern regarding Marilyn's unsteady gait, states she "does not meet criteria for release," and appears unfamiliar with her baseline functional status. You then called Marilyn's daughter and discussed the risks and benefits of discontinuing olanzapine and starting scheduled low dose risperidone with as needed IM haloperidol for acute agitation. You discussed your concerns regarding the anticholinergic burden of olanzapine and its likely contribution to Marilyn's delirium as well as her urinary retention. You reviewed the potential side effects of risperidone and haloperidol along with the evidence for their use in delirium.

Her daughter was not aware that the quetiapine had been discontinued and scheduled olanzapine was started. She was angry that she hadn't been notified of the changes but agreed to the additional changes you were recommending. You called the intern on the teaching service covering Marilyn and explained the medication changes you were making and the rationale. The intern wanted to know why you weren't referring Marilyn to geriatric psychiatry as "this is obviously a psychiatric issue at this point" because her antibiotic treatment for her UTI is nearly complete. You explain that delirium is an acute medical condition, and in the case of Marilyn, is likely caused by the ongoing sequelae of her UTI, the effects of the numerous antipsychotic agents she has been given in the hospital, and her prolonged period of immobility due to the fear of her falling and getting injured in the hospital. You reinforce that at the time, you are unable to assess for any underlying psychiatric disorders or neurocognitive impairment because of Marilyn's ongoing delirium. The two of you then discuss strategies to attempt to cease the use of the net-enclosure bed. The intern acknowledges that either the primary team or the night hospitalist providing cross coverage re-orders it every day when the nurses ask for it. They feel uncomfortable declining to write the order as the nurses feel they need it to keep Marilyn safe from falling.

The following day you receive a call from the registered nurse care manager (RNCM) asking why Marilyn isn't being referred to geriatric psychiatry as her ALF requested. You refer her to your note from the previous day and explain your rationale. She verbalizes understanding and states she will follow up with the facility. She calls back later in the day asking whether you can't adjust Marilyn's medications further to "get her out of the net-enclosure bed" because she can't be placed when she is in it. She also reported that the facility recommended that you order a cream from a compounding pharmacy that has halo-peridol, diphenhydramine, and lorazepam in it that staff can rub on Marilyn's hands or neck when she becomes agitated. You again refer the RNCM to your note from yesterday regarding medication chang-es and the rationale for them and decline to order the cream.

The following week, Marilyn is more alert, she is no longer retaining urine, and her delirium is improving though she continues to have waxing and waning orientation, mentation, and attention. She con-tinues to deny that she lives in an ALF and requests to return to her home. Her sleep-wake cycle is improved, though not yet near her baseline. She has not had behavioral dyscontrol or required any prn medication for agitation in over 72 hours. However, she remains in a net-enclosure bed. She is now a two-person assist with a front-wheel walker when ambulating and is being fed by nursing staff. The RNCM calls asking what you can do to get her out of the net-enclosure bed and mentions that her ALF cannot provide a two-person assist, nor can most memory care units. The RNCM is worried that an SNF won't accept Marilyn because of the behavioral issues she displayed earlier in her hospitalization. You tell the RNCM that you don't know what else to do but that you will talk to the primary team about ordering physical therapy and occupational therapy to work with Marilyn to see how they can help with restoration of her func-tional and cognitive abilities. You feel that the interventions required to keep Marilyn safe from falling, as well as the staff safe from her combative behavior that resulted from her delirium, have led to a de-cline in her condition despite your best efforts to treat her presenting problems.

Consider:

  1. Identify the ethical concerns with this situation.

2. What information will you need before a responsible decision can be made? (Consider what the information is and where it will come from.)

3. Who are stakeholders involved in the decision, and what is the process in which those involved could come to a decision (e.g., what tools are/could be used to create an informed decision)?

4. What are the values relevant to this problem? *Values* are the things that you believe are important in making the decision. They (should) determine priorities. Values relevant to this problem may not be representative of your own personal values or moral framework.

5. What are the options for the decision? Think in terms of values and feasibility (e.g., financial, political, organizational, religious constraints).

Marilyn Case Study Part Two

You are the FNP who was initially attending on Marilyn, but you have been covering different services for the last month. Marilyn was added back to your service today because it was felt she was no longer appropriate for the teaching service, as there are no active medical issues and she is awaiting disposition. She has now been hospitalized for over a month and remains in a net-enclosure bed. The psychiatric consultation liaison team has signed off as there were no acute psychiatric issues to address. They recommended tapering Marilyn's scheduled risperidone from 0.25mg twice daily and stopping it as her behavior tolerates because long-term use of antipsychotics is not recommended for the management of dementia. In reviewing the events of her hospitalization, you see that Marilyn had been out of the net-enclosure bed for two days but was placed back in it when she tripped over her pajama pants while walking unassisted to the bathroom and fell. She had gotten up, the bed alarm went off, and she fell before nursing staff responded to the bed alarm. Her pants were observed to be too long as she is quite petite. Marilyn was not injured when she fell. You are frustrated that she is back in a net-enclosure bed as you are concerned it will contribute to further deconditioning and make disposition even more challenging. She remains on B-12 replacement. Her CBC and CMP are normal, and her food and fluid intake is somewhat improved, though she continues to require nursing assistance with eating. Approximately one week after completing her antibiotics, occupational therapy completed cognitive testing with her using the St. Louis University Mental Status examination where she scored a 19, which is consistent with "dementia" but not diagnostic. You are unsure whether this represents her true baseline due to the confounding factors of recent UTI, delirium from infections and metabolic etiologies, and her prolonged hospitalization. You elect to start donepezil for dementia and begin tapering the risperidone as recommended. You try talking with the bedside nurse regarding the net-enclosure bed, but they respond, "I'm just a traveler."

Consider:

1. Identify the ethical concerns with this situation.

2. What information will you need before a responsible decision can be made? (Consider what the information is and where it will come from.)

3. Who are stakeholders involved in the decision, and what is the process in which those involved could come to a decision (e.g., what tools are/could be used to create an informed decision)?

4. What are the values relevant to this problem? *Values* are the things that you believe are important in making the decision. They (should) determine priorities. Values relevant to this problem may not be representative of your own personal values or moral framework.

5. What are the options for the decision? Think in terms of values and feasibility (e.g., financial, political, organizational, religious constraints).

Management of Case Studies

After all considerations, write a short narrative of how you believe is the best way to manage these situations; list core values important to you for managing the situation.

References

Derscheid, D. J., Lohse, C., & Arnetz, J. E. (2021). Risk factors for assault and physical aggression among medically hospitalized adult patients who had a behavioral emergency call: A descriptive study. *Journal of the American Psychiatric Nurses Association*, *27*(2), 99–110. https://doi.org/10.1177/1078390320983441

Ghosh, M., Twigg, D., Kutzer, Y., Towell-Barnard, A., De Jong, G., & Dodds, M. (2019). The validity and utility of violence risk assessment tools to predict patient violence in acute care settings: An integrative literature review. *International Journal of Mental Health Nursing*, *28*(6), 1248–1267. https://doi.org/10.1111/inm.12645

Haynes, T., & Pratt, E. S. (2009). Bed enclosures: Suitable safety net? *Nursing Management*, *40*(12), 36–39. https://doi.org/10.1097/01.numa.0000365470.32216.c3

Hicks, D. (2015). Can rounding reduce patient falls in acute care? An integrative literature review. *MEDSURG Nursing*, *24*(1), 51–55.

Inouye, S. K., Brown, C. J., & Tinetti, M. E. (2009). Medicare nonpayment, hospital falls, and unintended consequences. *New England Journal of Medicine*, *360*(23), 2390–2393. https://doi.org/10.1056/nejmp0900963

Lembitz, A., & Clarke, T. J. (2009). Clarifying "never events" and introducing "always events." *Patient Safety in Surgery*, *3*(1), 26. https://doi.org/10.1186/1754-9493-3-26

Maldonado, J. R. (2017). Acute brain failure: Pathophysiology, diagnosis, management, and sequelae of delirium. *Critical Care Clinics*, *33*(3), 461–519. https://doi.org/10.1016/j.ccc.2017.03.013

Moore, A., & Geist, R. (2015, May). Keeping patients safe from falls and pressure ulcers: In your patient advocate role, push for hospital policies that help prevent these "never events." *American Nurse Today*, *10*(5), 14–17.

Nawaz, H., Abbas, A., Sarfraz, A., Slade, M. D., Calvocoressi, L., Wild, D. G., & Tessier-Sherman, B. (2007). A randomized clinical trial to compare the use of safety net enclosures with standard restraints in agitated hospitalized patients. *Journal of Hospital Medicine*, 2(6), 385–393. https://shmpublications. onlinelibrary.wiley.com/doi/abs/10.1002/jhm.273

Peterson, C., Xu, L., & Florence, C. (2021). Average medical cost of fatal and non-fatal injuries by type in the USA. *Injury Prevention*, 27(1), 24–33. https:// doi.org/10.1136/injuryprev-2019-043544

Rowan, L., & Veenema, T. (2017). Decreasing falls in acute care medical patients. *Journal of Nursing Care Quality*, 32(4), 340–347. https://doi.org/10.1097/ ncq.0000000000000244

Sillner, A. Y., Holle, C. L., & Rudolph, J. L. (2019). The overlap between falls and delirium in hospitalized older adults. *Clinics in Geriatric Medicine*, 35(2), 221–236. https://doi.org/10.1016/j.cger.2019.01.004

TELEHEALTH

Telehealth is the use of technology-based virtual platforms to deliver care to patients. This care can include health information, prevention, monitoring, diagnosing, and delivering medical/nursing care. The three methods of providing telehealth are synchronous (delivery that occurs in real-time), asynchronous (collecting data that are then sent to a provider for review), and remote patient monitoring (utilizing technology capable of monitoring patient conditions; Mechanic et al., 2021).

The role of the nurse in providing telehealth services is as old as the telephone itself (Rutledge & Gustin, 2021). Nurses have provided advice, education, and support for patients via phone, internet, and other telecommunication devices as part of the continuity of care that the profession is committed to. While a convenience that none of us can imagine working without, telecommunication as a method for providing nursing care is not without challenges. Barriers to reimbursement, regulatory and licensing issues, and the technology itself often prevent nurses from feeling successful in utilizing telehealth. Nonetheless, telehealth is a tool that has allowed nurses to deliver care remotely, leading to improved access to healthcare for many, especially those in rural locations (Hoffman, 2020). There are many opportunities for expansion of telehealth and much work to be done to increase access through better broadband connectivity, addressing inequities that prevent utilization of telehealth, and overcoming adoption reluctance. Additionally, nursing education needs to expand to include the role of telehealth in academic programs. The COVID-19 pandemic ushered in a new level of adoption to telehealth practice and highlighted areas for improvement, including a closer examination of ethical practice in the virtual medical office.

Nurses face daily ethical challenges in delivering patient care. Practicing in the telehealth environment creates even more ethical issues for consideration. In fact, telehealth nursing may be one of the most complicated practice areas today and can be fraught with moral concern and uncertainty. Role conflict and inconsistent organizational policies can create frustration and add to job dissatisfaction and compassion fatigue already encountered by much of today's nursing workforce (Rutenberg & Oberle, 2008). The American Nurses Association (ANA) has recognized the unique challenges in delivering nursing care via telehealth in the Core Principles on Connected Health (2019). In this document, they have outlined 13 principles to provide guidance and emphasize that connected health technologies do not alter the standards of professional practice, and those nurses are still responsible for providing high-quality, lawful, evidence-based care grounded in the Code of Ethics for Nurses (ANA, 2015). In fact, principles of ethics may be even more crucial in the telehealth nursing specialty because of the remote contact (Rutenberg & Oberle, 2008). Regardless of the setting, nurses need to be able to identify sources of ethical distress and have a framework for evaluating an ethical course of action. If they are not able to do this, they are likely to experience increasing frustration, dissatisfaction, compassion fatigue, and burnout.

Case Study: Urgent Referrals in Telehealth

In the United States, more than 750,000 strokes occur in a year, and stroke is a leading cause of death due to cardiovascular disease (CDC, n.d.). Between 2017 and 2018, the costs to the healthcare system were close to $53 billion (CDC, n.d.). The consequences of stroke can be significant, with long-term disability including mobility issues (CDC, n.d.). There are early warning signs and symptoms of stroke that can increase survival, but knowledge of warning signs and risk factors still remains poor (Powers et al., 2019). Use of the emergency medical system is associated with a more rapid evaluation and treatment of stroke (Ekundayo, et al., 2013).

You are a primary care family nurse practitioner (FNP) providing synchronous telehealth care to an established patient. The patient, Robert, has requested a same day virtual appointment with a new onset of dizziness and facial weakness. Robert is a 57-year-old Caucasian male with mild hypertension who has been managed successfully with a daily beta blocker. You have not seen the patient in eight months, but at his last office visit he had normal labs including CBC, chem panel, and fasting cholesterol. The patient does have a strong family history of hypertension in both parents. His father died at age 72 from a cardiac event, and his mother died of metastatic breast cancer at age 68. The patient has admitted to a sedentary lifestyle. You log on to the visit to see Robert on your computer screen and immediately notice the left side of his face is drooping. You begin asking him questions about the onset of these new symptoms and notice that his speech is slightly slurred. At this point in the visit, you inform Robert that you are concerned about his symptoms and cannot rule out that he may have had a stroke. You advise that he needs to be seen in person for further evaluation and that you want to call an ambulance for him to be transported to the emergency department. The patient becomes visibly upset and states he is "not going to any damn hospital." You gently advise him that there are medications to treat stroke symptoms if given in a timely manner and that you are unable to provide care for his symptoms via a virtual format. He shouts that he is not going to the hospital and abruptly ends the visit.

Consider:

1. Identify the ethical concerns with this situation.

2. What information will you need before a responsible decision can be made? (Consider what the information is and where it will come from.)

3. Who are stakeholders involved in the decision, and what is the process in which those involved could come to a decision (e.g., what tools are/could be used to create an informed decision)?

4. What are the values relevant to this problem? *Values* are the things that you believe are important in making the decision. They (should) determine priorities. Values relevant to this problem may not be representative of your own personal values or moral framework.

5. What are the options for the decision? Think in terms of values and feasibility (e.g., financial, political, organizational, religious constraints).

Case Study: Time Management in Telehealth

You are the nurse in a primary care setting that often utilizes telehealth as a means for connecting with patients. During this shift, you are connected virtually to a well-known clinic patient who has a long list of diagnoses including severe depression and anxiety. The patient, Alice, is a 72-year-old woman who has recently been widowed. She has been treating her anxiety for two decades with as-needed alprazolam and, after the recent death of her husband, has also been started on a selective serotonin reuptake inhibitor. Alice is requesting a virtual visit today to "connect" about concerns. Your virtual clinic day is full, with a patient visit scheduled every 15 minutes. The clinic policy/ practice is to limit calls to 15 minutes and reschedule patients if they need more time. It is routine for the clinic management to discipline staff who do not adhere to the 15-minute appointment schedule. When you log on you can see that Alice appears somewhat disheveled in appearance, has rapid speech, and seems visually anxious. She proceeds to tell you that she is very concerned about the people who are in her house. When questioned, she cannot tell you who the people are or what they are doing there. She also tells you that she "doesn't always see them." She becomes tearful and tells you that she is scared and lonely and misses her husband. She states she "doesn't know what to do." When questioned she cannot tell you when she last ate or slept. You quickly realize that she needs more attention than you are going to be able to provide in a 15-minute visit. The 15-minute appointment time is up, and you need to end the visit to get to the next patient.

Consider:

1. Identify the ethical concerns with this situation.

2. What information will you need before a responsible decision can be made? (Consider what the information is and where it will come from.)

3. Who are stakeholders involved in the decision, and what is the process in which those involved could come to a decision (e.g., what tools are/could be used to create an informed decision)?

4. What are the values relevant to this problem? *Values* are the things that you believe are important in making the decision. They (should) determine priorities. Values relevant to this problem may not be representative of your own personal values or moral framework.

5. What are the options for the decision? Think in terms of values and feasibility (e.g., financial, political, organizational, religious constraints).

Case Study: Pharmaceutical Management Across Prescribing Boundaries

You are a primary care FNP providing synchronous telehealth. Your first virtual visit is with a well-established patient, Rosie, who is requesting a visit for medication refill. Rosie is a 37-year-old female with a lifelong seizure disorder who is on several anti-seizure medications due to frequent breakthrough seizures. She is not able to drive due to the frequency and severity of her seizure disorder. She also requires help with many of her day-to-day activities and has a live-in caregiver. When you connect for the virtual visit with Rosie, she tells you that she is calling from another state where she is visiting family, and her caregiver is not with her. She needs a refill on her seizure medications. In fact, she took the last dose yesterday and will need a new prescription called in as soon as possible to keep her blood concentrations within range to avoid a seizure. You are not a licensed practitioner in the state she is currently visiting.

Consider:

1. Identify the ethical concerns with this situation.

2. What information will you need before a responsible decision can be made? (Consider what the information is and where it will come from.)

3. Who are stakeholders involved in the decision, and what is the process in which those involved could come to a decision (e.g., what tools are/could be used to create an informed decision)?

4. What are the values relevant to this problem? *Values* are the things that you believe are important in making the decision. They (should) determine priorities. Values relevant to this problem may not be representative of your own personal values or moral framework.

5. What are the options for the decision? Think in terms of values and feasibility (e.g., financial, political, organizational, religious constraints).

Management of Case Studies

After all considerations, write a short narrative of how you believe is the best way to manage these situations; list core values important to you for managing each situation.

References

American Nurses Association. (2015). *Code of ethics for nurses with interpretive statements.* https://www.nursingworld.org/practice-policy/nursing-excellence/ethics/code-of-ethics-for-nurses/coe-view-only/

American Nurses Association. (2019). *ANA core principles on connected health.* https://www.nursingworld.org/~4a9307/globalassets/docs/ana/practice/ana-core-principles-on-connected-health.pdf

Centers for Disease Control and Prevention. (n.d.). *Stroke.* https://www.cdc.gov/stroke/facts.htm

Ekundayo, O. J., Saver, J. L., Fonarow, G. C., Schwamm, L.H., Xain, Y., Zhao, X., Hernandez, A. F., Peterson, E. D., & Cheng, E. M. (2013). Patterns of emergency medical services use and its association with timely stroke treatment findings from Get With the Guidelines – Stroke. *Circulation: Cardiovascular Quality and Outcomes, 6*(3), 262–269.

Hoffman, D. A. (2020). Increasing access to care: Telehealth during COVID-19. *Journal of Law and the Biosciences, 7*(1), 1–15. https://doi.org/10.1093/jlb/lsaa043

Mechanic, O. J., Persaud, Y., & Kimball, A. B. (2021). *Telehealth systems.* StatPearls Publishing. https://www.ncbi.nlm.nih.gov/books/NBK459384/

Powers, W. J., Rabinstein, M. D., Ackerson, T., Adeoye, O. M., Bambakidis, N. C., Becker, K., Biller, J., Brown, M., Demaerschalk, B. M., Hoh, B., Jauch, E. C., Kidwell, C. S., Leslie-Mazwi, T. M., Ovbiagele, B., Scott, P. A., Sheth, K. N., Southerland, A. M., Summers, D. V., & Tirschwell, D. L. (2019). Guidelines for the early management of patients with acute ischemic stroke: 2019 update to the 2018 guidelines for the early management of acute ischemic stroke: A guideline for healthcare professionals from the American Heart Association/American Stroke Association. *Stroke, 50*(12), e344–e418.

19

Rutenberg, C., & Oberle, K. (2008). Ethics in telehealth nursing practice. *Home Health Care Management & Practice, 20*(4), 342–348. https://doi.org/10.1177/1084822307310766

Rutledge, C. M., & Gustin, T. (2021). Preparing nurses for roles in telehealth: Now is the time! *Online Journal of Issues in Nursing, 26*(1). https://doi.org/10.3912/OJIN.Vol26No01Man03

GUIDING A SCHOOL OF NURSING THROUGH COVID-19 FOCUSING ON CLINICAL PLACEMENTS

Leading a school of nursing is a multifaceted and complex assignment in the best of times, rife with decisions potentially impacting generations of nurses. During extraordinary times such as COVID-19, these decisions become more intricate, and the process to make leadership decisions has many potential pitfalls for ethical dilemmas. Navigating these astonishing times while keeping nursing students, faculty, clinical partners, and patients safe amid the unknowns of COVID-19 requires a refined awareness of ethical dilemmas as well as a solid process for determining resolutions.

During the early days of COVID-19, in the spring of 2020 before COVID-19 vaccines were available for healthcare staff and students, the decision concerning keeping students in clinical practice or pulling them out for their safety was paramount and involved discussion with executive nurse leaders (C. Shillam, personal communication, November 17, 2021). According to Casey Shillam, Dean of the School of Nursing at the University of Portland, on one hand, the institution had an obligation to support students in their nursing programs and to continue their educational paths. Within a month of the outbreak of the pandemic, institutes of higher education had students scheduled to graduate from both undergraduate and graduate programs. The implications of pulling students out of clinical rotations would have disrupted not only their personal education pathways but also the nursing pipeline of new nursing graduates who were desperately needed on the frontlines of healthcare. Executive leaders had to weigh the nation's healthcare needs with the safety of their students (personal communication, November 17, 2021).

Points to consider during the early pandemic included the vast unknowns surrounding the virus, its transmission, and long-term impact on health. Additionally, there was not enough personal protective equipment (PPE), hesitancy on the side of clinical partners not wanting to have the added burden of students coming into clinical settings, especially in April, and questioning whether graduating nursing students had enough knowledge, skills, and experience to be safe. Multiple and distinct factors influenced the decision to pull students out of the undergraduate pre-licensure program as well as community-based clinical settings. There were not enough nursing faculty and preceptors to monitor the students during this time. The cost/benefit of having students in the community-based settings at a time when so much about the virus was unknown was not worth having students continue in community-based settings. The immediate result was a pause in nursing seniors about to graduate. This provided the health systems time and opportunity to determine:

- Is it feasible to have students in the health system?

- Who is providing and receiving the PPE? Is the school? Is the system?

- How are schools and clinical settings ensuring students' safety?

- What are State Board of Nursing guidelines and regulations regarding academic practice?

The guiding goal to these time-sensitive decisions was the risk/benefit ratio of student safety and patient and healthcare needs, balanced with the unknown and constantly changing chaos of the pandemic. The approach was systematic and followed an ethical framework that considered stakeholders, faculty members, students, and regulatory bodies (C. Shillam, personal communication, November 17, 2021).

Consider:

1. Identify the ethical concerns with this situation.

2. What information will you need before a responsible decision can be made? (Consider what the information is and where it will come from.)

3. Who are stakeholders involved in the decision, and what is the process in which those involved could come to a decision (e.g., what tools are/could be used to create an informed decision)?

4. What are the values relevant to this problem? *Values* are the things that you believe are important in making the decision. They (should) determine priorities. Values relevant to this problem may not be representative of your own personal values or moral framework.

5. What are the options for the decision? Think in terms of values and feasibility (e.g., financial, political, organizational, religious constraints).

Management of Case Study

After all considerations, write a short narrative of how you believe is the best way to manage this situation; list core values important to you for managing the situation.

20

EMERGENCY DEPARTMENT CLOSURE DECISION-MAKING: HEALTH SYSTEM AND COMMUNITY IMPACT

You are an APRN working in the C-suite of a not-for-profit health-care network, *Healthy*. Prior to your current position as Chief Clinical Operations Officer, you were a highly competent point-of-care provider and a vice-president clinical leader in the *Healthy* system. Your organization is the region's only level II adult trauma center and pediatric level II trauma center with a dedicated children's hospital. The surrounding acute care facilities are designated trauma level III and level IV. The nearest level I trauma center is 2.5 hours driving and 1.5 hours by helicopter.

The emergency department (ED) medical director and nursing director approach you regarding implementing an ambulance diversion program to temporarily close the ED to ambulance traffic during periods of ED saturation due to overcrowding or limited staffing resources. Both emergency leaders indicate that for more than a year the ED has been implementing a continuous quality improvement, evidence-based patient throughput plan, but at this point, the need is to implement an ambulance diversion program. The almost daily ED saturation is stressing the entire healthcare system.

Emergency medical services (EMS) is considered the junction between "health care, public health and public safety" (National Highway Traffic Safety Administration, n.d., para. 5). Demand for EMS is growing (Giannouchos et al., 2019). EMS consist of coordinated pre-hospital care and transport of a patient experiencing a medical emergency to an emergency receiving facility (Wilson et al., 2015). EMS are primarily delivered by ambulances equipped with lifesaving personnel and equipment (US Department of Transportation, 2015). EMS and emergency receiving facilities are tightly coupled systems dependent on each other. Tightly coupled systems are destabilized by pressures and failures that exceed the totality of the system's capabilities.

Optimizing operations for one section of a system arguably improves the performance of the entire system. Conversely, modifying structural paths in a system without replacement creates gaps and barriers in system performance. Broadly, periodic closure of an ED to ambulance traffic is a pathway change that has been associated with healthcare outcome deterioration, most likely due to delays in care (Hsuan et al., 2019). Patient-centric care (Gluyas, 2015) is not achieved in a system that does not provide timely, safe, effective, efficient, and equitable care. Temporary ED closures result in patients transported to locations that are potentially distant from family and the service area of the patient's provider.

Meeting Reporting Requirements Case Study

ED diversions present an ethical dilemma (Adkins & Werman, 2015; Geiderman et al., 2015; Nakajima & Vilke, 2015). There is no universal standard for temporary closure of an ED. The conditions under which an organization implements ambulance diversion vary. Temporary closure of an ED results in consequences to the individual patient and consequences to the community.

The EMS is designed with the purpose to reduce all-cause morbidity and mortality. Temporary closures of EDs result in delays in providing a range of interventions and services to the EMS catchment population. Ambulance offload delay (AOD) occurs when there is a prolonged delay of transferring a patient from an ambulance to an emergency receiving department. AOD literature has reported compromises in diagnosis and treatment of illness or injury survivors (Li et al., 2019). Ambulance diversion may temporarily relieve the overcrowding in the ED, but the AODs compound into larger complications for the community. It is well documented in the literature that ED saturation disproportionally impacts minority populations (Hsia et al., 2012; Hsia et al., 2017).

Healthy is in a crisis situation. Daily ED volume is significantly threatening the well-being of in-house patients and staff and threatening to harm the community at large. The organization has been implementing strategies to maximize patient flow for over a year involving interdisciplinary, interprofessional, and interdepartmental modeling using Lean/Toyota Production System approaches. However, the efficiency improvement gains have been swamped by an increase in ED annual volume of 3.56%, or approximately 20 patients per day. In addition, the demand for patient care providers and the *Healthy* position vacancy rate have continued to increase over the last year. The healthcare staffing shortage is not exclusive to *Healthy* but a national problem, as described in a plethora of articles.

Healthcare professionals have a fiduciary duty (American Nurses Association [ANA], 2015, Provision 2) to act in the best interest of a person, which may be an individual, family, group, community, or population. The person's interests are paramount. Provision 3 of the nursing Code of Ethics addresses keeping persons safe (ANA, 2015). The shortage of point-of-care providers makes the provisions of the Code of Ethics increasingly challenging to maintain. The problem of demand for ED services and availability of ED patient-centered services is not expected to improve soon. The ED personnel know the appropriate care to render to patients but due to constrained resources are not able to take all the actions appropriate to patient-centered care. This is creating moral distress affecting the department, which is rippling across the organization.

Consider:

1. Identify the ethical concerns with this situation.

2. What information will you need before a responsible decision can be made? (Consider what the information is and where it will come from.)

3. Who are stakeholders involved in the decision, and what is the process in which those involved could come to a decision (e.g., what tools are/could be used to create an informed decision)?

4. What are the values relevant to this problem? *Values* are the things that you believe are important in making the decision. They (should) determine priorities. Values relevant to this problem may not be representative of your own personal values or moral framework.

5. What are the options for the decision? Think in terms of values and feasibility (e.g., financial, political, organizational, religious constraints).

Management of Case Study

After all considerations, write a short narrative of how you believe is the best way to manage this situation; list core values important to you for managing the situation.

References

Adkins, E. J., & Werman, H. A. (2015). Ambulance diversion: Ethical dilemma and necessary evil. *American Journal of Emergency Medicine, 33*, 820–821. http://dx.doi.org/10.1016/j.ajem.2015.03.007

American Nurses Association. (2015). *Code of ethics for nurses with interpretive statements*. American Nurses Publishing.

Geiderman, J. M., Marco, C. A., Moskop, J. C., Adams, J., & Derse, A. R. (2015). Ethics of ambulance diversion. *American Journal of Emergency Medicine, 33*, 822–827. http://dx.doi.org/10.1016/j.ajem.2014.12.002

Giannouchos, T. V., Kum, H., Foster, M. J., & Ohsfeldt, R. L. (2019). Characteristics and predictors of adult frequent emergency department users in the United States: A systematic literature review. *Journal of Evaluation in Clinical Practice, 25*, 420–433. https://doi.org/10.1111/jep.13137

Gluyas, H. (2015). Patient-centred care: Improving health care outcomes. *Nursing Standard, 30*(4), 50–59. https://doi.org/10.7748/ns.30.4.50.e10186

Hsia, R. Y., Asch, S. M., Weiss, R. E., Zingmond, D., Liang, L. J., Han, W., McCreath, H., & Sun B. C. (2012). California hospitals serving large minority populations were more likely than others to employ ambulance diversion. *Health Affairs, 31*(8), 1767–1776. https://doi.org/10.1377/hlthaff.2011.1020

Hsia, R. Y., Sarkar, N., & Shen, Y. C. (2017). Impact of ambulance diversion: Black patients with acute myocardial infarction had higher mortality than whites. *Health Affairs, 36*(6), 1070–1078. https://www.doi.org/10.1377/hlthaff.2016.0925

Hsuan, C., Hsia, R. Y., Horwitz, J. R., Ponce, N. A., Rice, T., & Needleman, J. (2019). Ambulance diversions following public hospital emergency department closures. *Health Services Research, 54*, 870–879. https://doi.org/10.1111/1475-6773.13147

Li, M., Vanberkel, P., & Cater, A. J. (2019). A review on ambulance offload delay literature. *Health Care Management Science, 22*, 658–675. https://doi.org/10.1007/s10729-018-9450-x

Nakajima, Y., & Vilke, G. M. (2015). Ambulance diversion: The con perspective. *American Journal of Emergency Medicine, 33*, 818–819. https://www.ajemjournal.com/article/S0735-6757(15)00149-7/fulltext

National Highway Traffic Safety Administration. (n.d.). *What is EMS?* https://www.ems.gov/whatisems.html

US Department of Transportation. (2015). *Emergency medical services.* https://www.transportation.gov/careers/veterans/emergency-medical-services

Wilson, M. H., Habig, K., Wright, C., Hughes, A., Davies, G., & Imray, C. (2015). Pre-hospital emergency medicine. *Lancet, 386*(10012), 2526–2534. https://doi.org/10.1016/S0140-6736(15)00985-X

ETHICAL DILEMMAS IN SCHOOL OF NURSING LEADERSHIP PRE-COVID-19

Leadership in schools of nursing in pre-COVID-19 times certainly had unique-to-nursing challenges and ethical dilemmas. Some of those challenges included issues surrounding admissions, student retention, student progression, and student dismissal. Routinely, early in the admissions process, leadership in schools of nursing would feel pressure from institutional sources to admit or give an advantage to one applicant over another due to ties to the institution (J. Moceri, personal communication, November 22, 2021). In clinical settings, this can be likened to perhaps a staff member, a faculty member, a team member, or a patient asking for special treatment.

Ethical issues also arose around cumulative grade point averages (GPAs) and progression policies, especially concerning science and math standards. What were considerations for leadership in permitting students with borderline GPAs to progress? How did grade inflation affect these decisions? An example is a student with a 95.7 on their courses when 96 was passing. It is so close, and the institutional policy is not to round up. If an executive nurse leader were to pass the student in question, what would be the issues to consider? What about students who wanted to train as a caregiver but did not have the science and math background? In one institute of higher education, the decision was made to create a second major and minor in Integrative Health and Wellness to aid in the provision of alternative pathways to caregiving beyond nursing (J. Moceri, personal communication, November 22, 2021).

In addition to GPA, student behavior can be a catalyst for ethical dilemmas. In one instance, the student was not failing academically but had concerning and unprofessional behaviors. Leadership often needs to have difficult conversations with stakeholders, parents in this case, and determine best course of action to set up the student to be as successful as possible (J. Moceri, personal communication, November 22, 2021). Behavioral situations are often not clearly black and white due to the difficulties in qualifying and quantifying student behavior.

In addition to student issues, executive leadership are involved with faculty hiring, retention, and promotion in schools of nursing. Ethical concerns in this realm include how to determine who is hired and what rubric is created and applied equitably to minimize subjectivity (J. Moceri, personal communication, November 22, 2021). Once hired, what is the best way to provide support to retain and support faculty members? How are individuals' research trajectories supported evenly across programs and among DNP- and PhD-prepared faculty?

In all these scenarios, developing a standardized approach to identifying and resolving these dilemmas is paramount.

Consider:

1. Identify the ethical concerns with this situation.

2. What information will you need before a responsible decision can be made? (Consider what the information is and where it will come from.)

3. Who are stakeholders involved in the decision, and what is the process in which those involved could come to a decision (e.g., what tools are/could be used to create an informed decision)?

4. What are the values relevant to this problem? *Values* are the things that you believe are important in making the decision. They (should) determine priorities. Values relevant to this problem may not be representative of your own personal values or moral framework.

5. What are the options for the decision? Think in terms of values and feasibility (e.g., financial, political, organizational, religious constraints).

Management of Case Study

After all considerations, write a short narrative of how you believe is the best way to manage this situation; list core values important to you for managing the situation.

INDEX

B-C

CPSIA information can be obtained
at www.ICGtesting.com
Printed in the USA
BVHW032326290722
643339BV00004B/18

9 781646 480906